La Vida Loco

Surviving Long Covid with horrible fatigue and a worse attitude.

Alexia Daniels

Copyright © Alexia Daniels 2025. All rights reserved.

This book or any portion thereof may not be reproduced or used in any manner whatsoever without the express written permission of the publisher except for the use of brief quotations in a book review.

Any referenced to historical events, real people, or places are used fictitiously. Names, characters, and places are products of the author's imagination.

Printed in the United Kingdom.

First Printing , 2025

ISBN:- 978-1-0687840-2-6 (Paperback)

ISBN:- 978-1-0687840-3-3 (eBook)

Alexia Daniels

Southsea, Hampshire, UK.

contents

1. Dedication — 1
2. Introduction — 2
4. How To Use This Book Without Using Too Much Energy — 5
6. Part One - WTF Is This? — 9
7. Myths, Misinformation & The "It's All In Your Head" Brigade — 13
8. Vaccines, Long Covid, and That One Guy on Facebook — 16
9. Is it Long Covid or Just Life? — 21
10. Long Covid—It's Not All in Your Head (Though Some People Thought It Was) — 25
11. Medical Mayhem (Diagnosis) — 30
12. Part One - Summary For The Foggy. — 36
14. Part Two - WTF Do I Feel Like This? — 39

15.	Brain Fog - Damn, I Forgot What This Chapter Was About	42
16.	Breathing/ Dizziness and the Body	44
17.	The Brain, the Mood, and the Juddering Mess	51
18.	The Muscles, The Joints, and the Betrayal	57
19.	Gut Feelings	63
20.	The Weird and the Widespread	70
21.	Part Two - Summary For The Foggy	77
23.	Part Three - HTF Do I Live Now?	80
24.	Showering Without Weeping	83
25.	Cooking When Your Arms Feel Like Lead	85
26.	Cleaning Without Collapsing	87
27.	Managing Family Life When You Feel Like a Ghost	89
28.	Good Day / Bad Day Routines	91
29.	Part Three - Summary For The Foggy.	94
31.	Part Four - WTF Happened To Me?	97
32.	The Grief You Didn't Expect	101
33.	When It All Gets a Bit Much	105
34.	Fear, Reinfection, and the Eternal Internal Scream	113
35.	Asking for Help	118
36.	The Awkward Bit: When Others Don't Get It	122
37.	Who Am I Now? Identity and Chronic Illness	125
38.	The Role of the Patient	131
39.	God Forbid I Laugh	137

40.	Part Four - Summary For The Foggy.	141
42.	Part Five - WTF Do I Say?	145
43.	How to Explain Long Covid Without Screaming Into a Plant	150
44.	Conversations That Matter: Talking to Your People	155
45.	Talking to Your Boss and Colleagues	158
46.	Part Five - Summary For The Foggy.	160
48.	Part Six - HTF Do I Keep Going?	163
49.	Breathwork	166
50.	Siesta or Crash?	169
51.	The Boom and Bust Cycle	173
52.	A Diet That Won't Bankrupt You or Make You Smell of Kale	177
53.	Resting	183
54.	Energy Conservation	186
55.	Finding New Joy: Writing, Reading, Making Stuff (Badly, Brilliantly, or Just Because)	189
56.	Making Peace With Mobility Aids	194
57.	Finding calm in a nervous system that forgot how to calm down	197
58.	The Bare Minimum	202
59.	Making Your Home LoCo-Friendly (Without Re-designing It Like a Hospital)	207
60.	Part Six - Summary For The Foggy.	211
62.	Part Seven - WTF About the Future?	214

63.	Getting Help (Without Crying) on a Government Helpline	220
64.	Medication, Magic Pills...	226
65.	Relationships, Work and the Real World	236
66.	"How Are You Today/Now?" – The Daily Dilemma	238
67.	Small People Who Grow Up Fast	243
68.	Sex, Dating, and Other Things You're Too Tired For	246
69.	Occasions and Leaving the House	249
70.	Work	251
71.	Surviving Work With a Fluctuating Condition	256
72.	Part Seven - Summary For The Foggy.	264
74.	Part Eight - WTF About Money?	266
75.	Benefits and Bureaucratic Bingo	271
76.	Employment and Support Allowance (ESA)	273
77.	Universal Credit (UC): The Necessary Evil	275
78.	General Survival Tips for the Bureaucratic Maze	278
79.	Part Eight - Summary for the Foggy	281
81.	A Last Word From Your Friend on the Sofa	283
82.	About the Author	286
83.	Thank You	287
84.	Glossary	289
85.	Useful Stuff - Resources	293
86.	Useful Stuff - Fit Note Letter	295
87.	Useful Stuff - Workplace Adjustment Request Template	296

88. Useful Stuff - Tracker For GP   298

Dedication

This book is for you,
with all my love.

Introduction

Why This Book Exists

Long Covid is hard to explain, often invisible, and frequently misunderstood. Also, medical leaflets are boring and smell of waiting rooms. This book is a pep talk in paperback. It's the mate who texts you memes of a T-Rex trying to put a fitted sheet on a bed when you're feeling low. It's practical. It's funny. It tells you what is happening with your body and how to make peace with it (or at least negotiate a ceasefire).

We'll cover everything from pacing and breathing exercises to explaining to your boss that you're not bunking off; your mitochondria just gave up. This is all backed by science, real stories, and a refusal to sugar-coat anything unless it's medicinal chocolate.

Ground Rules

This isn't a substitute for medical advice. Use it as a supplement, like vitamin D, but with fewer side effects. Yes, if you read the blurb, I am a nurse, but this is about being firmly on the other side of the consulting room and my own experience and opinion. I don't speak here as a nurse, but I know many of you reading this might have picked Long Covid up through work, and for that, you have my respect, sympathy and love.

If you need urgent help, see a GP or visit a proper medical service, not a bloke on Facebook who sells magic beans. I'm not promising a cure. I'm promising solidarity, sarcasm, and some strategies that might help.

Now, let's get started because you deserve answers. I also need to make myself feel useful after forgetting what I walked into the room for—again. And a final thing – read this book in bits, dot about, ignore what doesn't work for you, and pour over the bits that do, but rest, take your time, and most importantly, allow yourself to laugh.

"They call it Long COVID — not because it lasts forever, but because it gives everyone else a long time to get very uncomfortable when I say I'm still sick."

HOW TO USE THIS BOOK WITHOUT USING TOO MUCH ENERGY

Congratulations! You've picked up (or possibly dropped and then picked up again) a book that promises to make you laugh *and* help you survive Long Covid. That's multitasking, which you should **not** be doing if you've got brain fog, so let's slow this down.

This is not a book to be read in one sitting unless you enjoy waking up three days later next to a half-eaten packet of oatcakes and wondering why your eyeballs feel fizzy.

1. Use the Book Like a Buffet

You don't need to start at Chapter One and march stoically forward. This book is like a tapas bar for your slightly frazzled nervous system. Dip in, pick what you fancy, and leave the rest for another day (or year).

There are:-

- Lots of spaces to keep eye strain to a minimum and so you can scribble notes and highlight things if needed.

- Summaries at the end of each chapter for the Foggy.

- Bullet Points to keep things simple.

- Your Friend on the Sofa offering a few words of support.

Craving a laugh? Head to the chapter with the most jokes, whichever it is. I've forgotten...Need a pep talk? There's one in here somewhere. Probably. Are you looking for tips on how to wash your hair without needing a lie-down afterwards? Yes, we went there.

2. Read in the Position of Your Choosing

Upright, reclined, horizontal, or folded into a blanket cocoon—we don't judge. If you can hold the book/phone/e-reader with your nose while your arms rest like deflated spaghetti, go for it.

Bonus points if you manage to read while inside a duvet fortress with a hot water bottle sidekick.

3. No Tests. No Homework. No Healing Pressure.

This isn't school. There's no pop quiz at the end. You are not obligated to implement **any** advice unless it genuinely sounds like something that won't make you worse. If your body's idea of exercise is shifting from one butt cheek to the other—great. Celebrate that win.

4. Use the Margins

Got a pencil? Scribble in the margins. Write your own responses, eye-rolls, or alternate titles (like "A Series of Unfortunate Symptoms").

Make it yours. Turn this book into your Long Covid sidekick, therapist, and emotional support gremlin.

5. Come Back Later
Brain not braining? Eyes doing that blurry nonsense again? No problem. Just shut the book and walk—no, **wobble**—away. It'll be here when you're ready. Possibly smugly, but it *will* be here.

6. Share with Caution
Feel like handing it to a well-meaning relative who just said, "Have you tried yoga?" Go ahead. Just be prepared that they may flip through it, chuckle nervously, and then quietly back away. It's a self-help book and a subtle weapon in the war against unsolicited advice.

Final Thought: This book is here to meet you where you are—even if where you are is under three blankets and next to a pile of clean laundry you may or may not ever put away. You're doing great. Pace yourself. Pick your pages. Laugh when you can. Rest when you must.

Welcome to the weird, wobbly, and wickedly honest ride.

"Having Long COVID is like being haunted by a virus that already dumped you —

but now it just lingers, ruins your life, and eats all your energy snacks."

Part One - WTF IS THIS?

I Survived Covid – So Why Do I Feel Like a Morris Minor has run Over me?

Picture this: you did everything right. Wore the mask. Got the jabs. Washed your hands like you were prepping for open-heart surgery (wore the bin bags when PPE was rarer than a quiet neighbour during lockdown). You even avoided hugging your nan for the better part of a year. Still, somehow, COVID found you like a heat-seeking missile of doom with an agenda — and no regard for personal boundaries. You recovered, or so you thought. The fever broke. The cough receded. The lateral flow tests stopped looking like a bar chart. You tried to go back to normal. But your body had other ideas. Now it's been weeks — or months — and you still feel like a hungover scarecrow mugged by gravity and possibly reversed over by a Morris Minor. In a cul-de-sac. Repeatedly. Welcome to the confusing, surreal, and often maddening world of post-viral syndromes — where your body lingers in a permanent state of "meh," your to-do list becomes a to-don't list, and your social battery has all the endurance of a wet crisp.

So What Is Long Covid, Then?

According to the NHS, Long COVID refers to symptoms that persist long after the initial infection and can't be explained by another diagnosis. It's like your body got bored with being healthy and decided to go off-script.

Symptoms include:

- Fatigue

    - *"Not just a bit tired," more like "I've been hit by a small lorry"*

- Brain fog

    - *"Good luck finishing a sentence without forgetting your name"*

- Breathlessness

    - *"Going upstairs now counts as cardio"*

- Palpitations

    - *"Your heart attending a '90s rave"*

- Muscle aches

    - *"Way beyond the normal 'ohh' of trying to get to your feet when you are over 40"*

- Anxiety and depression

    - *"Because, why not? It's all going a little runny."*

- Stomach and Bowel problems.
  - *"Yay"*

And a delightful carousel of other random oddities. (Who knew long COVID would make me lose my love of a good Chinese takeaway?)

It affects people differently. Some folks are back at work within weeks. Some months or years later, they still wonder why brushing their teeth leaves them feeling like they ran a marathon.

The Baffling Beast That Is Long Covid

Let's call a spade a spade: Long COVID-19 is confusing for patients, GPs, and scientists. It's like your immune system threw a tantrum during the pandemic and decided to keep sulking in the corner even long after the main event. Long COVID, or Post-COVID-19 Syndrome (if you're feeling fancy), or LoCo if you are like me, refers to symptoms that persist long after the initial infection—and crucially, they can't be explained by something else, like anaemia or the soul-sapping void of modern capitalism.

It's Not All in Your Head (Though Your Head Might Be Involved)

You are not imagining it. Your symptoms are real. And no, Karen, it's not just stress, gluten, or Mercury retrograde.Scientists suspect Long Covid results from multiple overlapping culprits, and this list changes daily.

The REACT study from Imperial College London estimated that over 2 million people in the UK alone were experiencing Long Covid symptoms. Two. Million. You're not rare. You're a founding member of one of the largest unrequested clubs in modern medical history.The big takeaway? This is new, and research is evolving every day. We can do more as we learn; you can be part of that.

Researchers believe it might be caused by:

- Immune system overreaction (your body goes into full DEFCON 1 and then forgets to stand down)

- Microclots (tiny clots that mess with oxygen delivery like a dodgy broadband connection)

- Autonomic nervous system dysfunction (your body forgets how to do automatic things like regulate heart rate or blood pressure)

- Lingering viral reservoirs (basically, Covid squatting in your tissues rent-free)

> **Your Friend On the Sofa**
>
> There isn't one cause, so it's been such a nightmare to research, diagnose and treat. But don't despair. You're not imagining it, you're not making it up, and no, essential oils are not the only answer, even if they smell lovely.

MYTHS, MISINFORMATION & THE "IT'S ALL IN YOUR HEAD" BRIGADE

Let's get something out of the way right now: **You did not cause this. You are not imagining it. And you are not alone.**

Long Covid is real. It is measurable. It is being studied globally. It's shown in blood tests, brain scans, and thousands of medical journals. And yet, despite all that, some people still want to believe it's... a vibe? A trend? A collective illusion?

Unfortunately, this condition has been haunted not just by symptoms, but by **misinformation**, **stigma**, and **some deeply unhelpful opinions from people who think reading one meme equals medical training**.

Let's walk through some of the greatest hits.

"Covid isn't real." / "It never happened."

You know what's weird? A global pandemic where over six million people died, and somehow, there are still folks out there saying, *"Did we overreact?"* No, Brenda. We did not. Covid did happen. It disrupted life, health systems, and economies on a global scale. People died.

People were disabled. People *are still being affected*. The fact that some want to pretend it was all an overblown cold is not just offensive — it's dangerous.

" It was made in a lab." / "It was designed on purpose."

Listen, the *origin* of the virus? Genuinely still being investigated. Scientists will probably be debating this for years. But here's the thing: **where it came from doesn't change the fact that it's here, it's real, and millions are still recovering from it.** Blaming shadowy forces doesn't help the people struggling to get through a shower without needing a nap. It's a distraction. It's not the point. Move on.

"You probably wouldn't be sick if you were healthier."

Ah, yes, the myth of the Perfect Immune System™, as if going for runs and juicing carrots makes you biologically untouchable. The truth? **Long Covid doesn't care how many steps you did or if you ate chia seeds**. It has affected marathon runners, Olympic athletes, vegans, teenagers, children, and people who've never touched a cigarette in their lives. This isn't about "healthy lifestyles." It's about a complex, unpredictable virus and the chaotic ways it can affect the body long-term.

"You must be exaggerating." / "It's just anxiety."

Ah, the classic. When medicine doesn't understand something, the fallback is often, *"Well, maybe it's psychological."* But this is not hysteria in a corset. This is not burnout. This is not attention-seeking. **This is a physical illness with biological roots** — affecting your vascular system, nervous system, immune function, and more. And yes, anxiety can *come with it*, but it is not *the cause*. Wouldn't *you* be anxious if your body suddenly stopped working as it used to?

"It's all in your head."

In a way, this one's funny — because **a lot of Long Covid *is* in the head...**It affects the *brain*, causing memory issues, cognitive dysfunction ("brain fog"), and inflammation that shows up on actual scans. But that's not what people mean when they say this. They mean: *"I can't see it, so it must not be real."*

We say you cannot see radio waves, **yet you still post conspiracy theories on WiFi.**

"Maybe you just don't want to get better."

Ah, the idea that people are choosing this. It is as if everyone with Long Covid is just deeply committed to a bit of light malingering. As if we *want* to lose jobs, miss out on life, spend our days rationing energy and explaining our illness like it's a customer service script.

> **Your Friend on the Sofa**
>
> Let's be very clear: **no one wants this.** No one enjoys it. We are not faking. We are not weak. We are not lazy. We are tired because we are sick. Not because we have a poor attitude.

Vaccines, Long Covid, and That One Guy on Facebook

Ah, vaccines. The tiny jab that launched a thousand conspiracy theories, WhatsApp group arguments, and at least one heated Christmas dinner that ended in someone storming out with the trifle.

Let's get one thing clear right out of the gate: **The COVID vaccine did not cause your Long Covid.**

Nope. Not even the booster. Not even the one that made your arm feel like it got punched by a moody kangaroo.

Let's Break Down the Myths (So We Can Set Fire to Them With Science)

Myth 1: "The vaccine gave me Long Covid."

Nope. Long Covid, by definition, requires you to have *had Covid* first. The vaccine? Not Covid. It's like saying you got a hangover from a cocktail umbrella. You may have gotten some side effects—fatigue, chills, a moment where you questioned all your life choices—but those are **short-term immune responses**, not a months-long chronic illness.

Please think of the vaccine like a drill sergeant yelling at your immune system to get it together. Sometimes it shouts a bit loud and leaves you with a fever, but it's prepping your body for battle, not causing a 12-week-long viral symphony in your mitochondria.

Myth 2: "Everyone with Long Covid had the vaccine first."

Also false. Many people with Long Covid caught the virus in the early days—before vaccines were even available, when the official advice was "Don't worry unless you're coughing up a lung while riding a unicycle."

In fact, the **majority of early Long Covid sufferers** were the ones begging for vaccines while sipping flat Lucozade and hallucinating episodes of *Antiques Roadshow*.

Myth 3: "The vaccine doesn't work because I got Covid anyway."

Vaccines aren't magic spells. They don't make you immune from catching Covid—they train your body to *handle it better*. Think of it like putting your immune system through a crash course called "How Not to Lose It When a Virus Shows Up Absolutely."

Still got Covid? Sure. But maybe instead of a hospital, you just got three days of watching Netflix in a dressing gown. That's a win.

So... Should I Get Another Vaccine If I Have Long Covid?

Here's where it gets *personal*. And nuanced. And not something your neighbour's brother's cat's TikTok doctor should be deciding.

- Some people with Long Covid **found vaccines helped**, even improved symptoms.

- Others **felt a temporary flare-up** of symptoms post-jab, or

- no change.

- And a few said, "Honestly, I'm just tired of being a human pin cushion," and opted out.

The important bit? **It's your choice.**

There's no one-size-fits-all answer, and that's okay. The goal is to work with a proper healthcare provider, not a bloke in a hoodie shouting into a YouTube livestream with a whiteboard and no qualifications.

A Note on Side Effects (Let's Be Honest)

Yes, vaccines can have side effects. Sore arms. Fevers. The overwhelming urge to tell strangers you've "just had your jab" like it's a new tattoo.

But Long Covid isn't one of them. You didn't "catch" chronic illness from the vaccine. If you've been feeling worse after it, it could be:

- A coincidental flare of your existing condition

- Your immune system is having a dramatic moment

- A late-onset Covid infection that was already brewing

Either way, don't let fear-mongering memes convince you your entire medical history began with a nurse and a plunger.

Final Thought

Vaccines aren't perfect. Medicine isn't ideal. However, misinformation is like giving your brain a virus with a Facebook logo. Protect yourself—yes, from COVID—but also from being dragged into the infinite swamp of "just asking questions" disguised as scientific inquiry.

You're allowed to be tired, cautious, and confused. But don't be misled. Long Covid is exhausting enough without debating strangers about spike proteins in a car park.

So Why Do These Myths Persist?

Long Covid challenges people's sense of safety. If illness is random and unpredictable, anyone could get sick — even them. That's uncomfortable. So they build stories to protect themselves. *You must have done something wrong. You must be different. You must have made it up.*

It's easier for them to judge than to sit with the truth: **this could happen to anyone.**

Here's What's True:
- Long Covid is not a moral failure.

- It is not punishment for poor choices.

- It is not your fault.

- It is not "society's sickness."

- And it is, absolutely, **not imaginary**.

Who spreads those myths? **They're wrong. Loud wrong. Compassion-deficient wrong.** And while anger is a valid response, try not to waste your precious energy fighting every internet stranger who reads one Insta post and thinks they're a virologist.

> **Your Friend on the Sofa**
>
> Hold on to the facts. Find your people. Share your story with those who listen. And remember: **you deserve support, not suspicion.**

IS IT LONG COVID OR JUST LIFE?

Yes, This Is Happening To You

You might be wondering if you're just a bit out of shape, or lazy, or depressed. You've been unwell, so of course you got a little unfit. Spoiler: you're not. Long Covid doesn't care how fit you were, whether you climbed mountains or only climbed into bed. It's not a failure of willpower. It's a physiological condition that needs respect, not self-blame. You were not somehow unworthy, you did not invite this in, you were just damn unlucky.

You, But On Hard Mode

One of the worst things about Long Covid is its invisibility. You may look normal(ish). You might even sound fine if someone calls during your one-hour clarity between 11 am and 12 pm on a Wednesday. But inside, it's a war zone. Your body is waging battles most people can't see. When you tell someone, "I'm still not better," they say, "But you look fine." You say, "I had a shower and needed to lie down for three hours," and they say, "Must be nice to rest." You cancel plans again, and they say, "You just need to push yourself." You resist the urge to launch a cushion across the room because a) you don't have the energy, and b) cushions are expensive.

How Do You Know If It's Long Covid?

You might be wondering: Is this still Covid? Is this anxiety? Is this just what ageing feels like? The answer: maybe all, maybe none. But here's when to get things checked:

> If it's been more than 12 weeks and you're still wiped out
>
> If your symptoms come and go like a dodgy WiFi connection
>
> If rest doesn't restore you
>
> If exertion makes things worse, not better

Your Friend on the Sofa

This book is not a cure, and I wish to heaven it were. It won't give you your old energy back. But it might give you a laugh. And a nudge. And a reminder that you are not alone. You are not weak. You are not making it up. You are surviving in the most frustrating, foggy, brilliant way possible. So if all you did today was read this lying down in a pair of trackies with biscuit crumbs on your chest, consider it a win. Long Covid is lonely. Fatigue makes socialising hard. Symptoms are invisible. People think you're just tired or overreacting. But there's a growing network of support online and off. Join groups, follow doctors and researchers on social media (for goodness' sake, check they are and haven't just bought a white jacket off Amazon or have a diploma in drinking urine) and most importantly: connect. You're not weak. You're not dramatic. You're ill. And you deserve to be believed, treated, and maybe even brought a biscuit occasionally. Now let's dive deeper.

What Is a Post-Viral Syndrome?

Imagine your body fighting off a virus. It throws everything at the invader—fever, fatigue, inflammation, the whole immune system circus. Eventually, the virus is cleared, the worst seems over, and everyone expects you to bounce back, sip some electrolytes, and get on with your life.

But you don't. Instead, your body keeps acting like it's still under attack. Someone forgot to switch off the emergency alarm system, and now it's just blaring 24/7 while your body stumbles around asking, *"Wait, are we still at war?"*

Welcome to the strange, glitchy world of **post-viral syndromes** — when your immune system throws a tantrum long after the virus has packed its bags, left the party, and deleted you from its contacts. You're not sick in the traditional "take paracetamol and wait a few days" way. You're stuck in a confusing aftermath, where your body feels buffering. Indefinitely.

It's like being ghosted by your health. You want answers. Your test results might say you're "fine." But your body says otherwise — in the form of crushing fatigue, brain fog, weird neurological symptoms, heart palpitations, shortness of breath, and a long list of other joys. It can feel like your body is trying to send an error report in a language no one's taught you to read.

But here's the important part: you are not imagining this. Post-viral illnesses are not new. They've been showing up quietly, inconveniently, for decades, after infections like Epstein-Barr virus (glandular fever/mono), dengue, SARS, Zika, Lyme disease, and even the flu.

They just haven't had a spotlight because, frankly, they're messy, hard to explain, and not very media-friendly.

They don't come with neat treatment plans or easy soundbites. You can't tie a ribbon around a post-viral syndrome and call it a comeback story. So they've often been dismissed, minimised, or flat-out ignored.

Enter Covid. And suddenly, this post-viral party has millions of uninvited guests — from every continent, background, and age group — all experiencing the same baffling symptoms. This is where *Long Covid* walks into the room with a dramatic sigh and a suitcase full of symptom spreadsheets.

Long COVID is a post-viral syndrome—a big one. Because of the pandemic's sheer scale, these illnesses have finally been pushed into the global conversation. It's like the world finally noticed the fire because the smoke got too thick to ignore.

And Remember - The Long Haul Isn't Linear

Recovery from Long COVID is not like climbing a staircase. It's more like being in a lift that's been sabotaged by a drunk raccoon. Some days you go up. Some days you plummet. Some days, you press a button that makes a weird noise, and nothing happens. That doesn't mean you're failing. It means you're living inside a body still recalibrating — or sulking. PEM (Post-Exertional Malaise) is the standout party crasher here. It's when doing something "normal" like hoovering, answering emails, or daring to think about exercise leads to a crash, hours or even days later. The crash is not a metaphor. It's a real, physiological backlash. Your mitochondria essentially call a strike.

LONG COVID—IT'S NOT ALL IN YOUR HEAD (THOUGH SOME PEOPLE THOUGHT IT WAS)

If you've ever mentioned "Long Covid" and been met with a blank stare, a confused eyebrow, or someone saying, "Is that still a thing?"—congratulations, you've experienced what early Long Covid sufferers went through **every single day** back in 2020.

Let's rewind, shall we?

In the Beginning: There Was The Virus, and Then... the Weird Hangover

When COVID-19 first burst onto the global scene like an uninvited guest with no regard for personal space, the general expectation was:

"You'll either get better in two weeks... or you won't be here to worry about it."

Charming, right?

But then something strange started happening.

A few weeks after "recovering," many people—many previously healthy, youngish, energetic types—began reporting something odd: **they weren't bouncing back**. They weren't dying, sure, but they weren't exactly alive and thriving either. They were... stuck. On pause. Like someone had unplugged them and forgotten where they put the charger.

Enter the Internet: The First Support Groups Were in the Wild

Medical experts hadn't quite caught on yet, but *patients* had. Support groups began springing up on Facebook, Reddit, and Twitter (back when it was still Twitter and not an abstract art project). People compared notes, ranted, cried, and coined "Long Covid."

It wasn't doctors who named it. It wasn't researchers. It was the *people living it*.

And that's important.

The Medical World Catches Up (Slowly, and With a Bit of Grumbling)

By mid-to-late 2020, the medical community grudgingly began to admit something weird was going on. Studies started trickling in. Clinics were set up (often badly), and scientists began asking, "Wait... what *is* this thing?"

It didn't fit nicely into existing boxes. It wasn't just post-viral fatigue. It wasn't mental illness (though it certainly made many people question their sanity). It was something new—or at least something newly *noticed*.

Slowly, Long Covid was acknowledged by:

- **The World Health Organisation**

- **The UK's NHS and NICE guidelines**

- **The US Centres for Disease Control (CDC)**

- ...and more governments than you'd expect, though fewer than you'd *hope*.

The result? It went from "random Facebook whinging" to a **recognised medical condition** with its own code and all the bureaucratic flair that entails.

Where Are We Now With Research?

We've moved from *"Is this even real?"* to *"How on earth does this work?"*

Here's where the research stands—boiled down into digestible bits, no medical degree required:

- **There's real money going into it** (finally). Major funding bodies like the NIH (US), NIHR (UK), and the EU are throwing millions at researchers like a medical game show.

- **There are hundreds of studies underway**, including brain scans, blood tests, and gut microbiome poking. A few scientists have definitely lost sleep over this (join the club).

- **Multiple theories are in play**: viral persistence, immune dysregulation, microclots, autonomic dysfunction, etc. The scientific community agrees it's real—they're just arguing about the *how* and *why*.

- **There's still no one-size-fits-all treatment**, but new trials are testing everything from antihistamines to antivirals to repurposed drugs that sound like rejected Marvel villains.

The truth is, science takes time. Especially when what you're studying is like trying to solve a Rubik's Cube while blindfolded, underwater, and being heckled by trolls on Twitter.

The Shift in Public Awareness

We've come a long way from:

"It's anxiety. Have you tried going for a jog?" to "We need national clinics, rehabilitation programs, and ongoing research funding."

(Not nearly far enough, but hey, progress.)

- Media coverage has improved (no more headlines like "COVID Lingers in Lazy People").

- More doctors are aware, though sadly, "aware" doesn't always equal "helpful."

- Celebrities and public figures are starting to speak up. (Let's be real: nothing says 'this is real' like a mildly famous person tweeting about it from their hyperbaric oxygen chamber.)

- Access to care is patchy at best.

- Some people are still dismissed, misdiagnosed, or given yoga leaflets and vibes.

- There's a persistent myth that vaccines "caused" Long Covid (spoiler: they didn't).

- And there's still a sense among many patients that they're left to manage this condition with little more than a notebook, a cup of tea, and a sense of humour held together with duct tape.

And Yet... We Still Have Work To Do

Medical Mayhem (Diagnosis)

When to See a GP (and How to Be Taken Seriously)

If you're still feeling like death warmed up, microwaved, and then forgotten on the side of the bed more than **12 weeks** after catching COVID, it's time to *book that GP appointment*. This is not just "a bit run down" anymore—this is your body throwing up a protest sign and refusing to attend the wellness rally.

Seeing a GP can feel like preparing for battle in a foggy swamp while wearing socks on your hands. But don't worry—I've got your back. Here's how to increase your chances of being taken seriously, heard, and ideally not prescribed a multivitamin and a patronising nod.

The NHS Is Great, Unless You're Trying to Get an Appointment

We love the NHS. We really do. But getting seen these days can feel like trying to book Glastonbury tickets on dial-up.

A Note on Expectations

The NHS is full of brilliant people working in an underfunded, overburdened system. Be kind, but be firm. You're not asking for special treatment. You're asking for basic care. And maybe a biscuit.

What to Expect from a Clinic

- Assessment: Someone will listen to you. Which is already a win.

- Support plans: Fatigue management, breathing exercises, pacing guides.

- Referrals: Maybe physio, maybe CBT (for coping, not because it's all in your head).It's not a silver bullet. But it's a start.

- If There's No Clinic Nearby (or the Waitlist Is Longer Than EastEnders)Self-management resources: Use NHS pages, charities like Long Covid Support, and pacing apps.

- Join support groups: Online ones are brilliant for tips, solidarity, and memes.

- Stay informed: Follow researchers and doctors who specialise in Long Covid. You'll feel less alone and more empowered.

Be Specific (Even If It's Weird)

Your GP is not a mind reader. They are also not psychic, omniscient, or, in most cases, especially experienced in Long COVID (yet). So help them out.

- **Write down your symptoms**, ideally in bullet points. Extra credit if you've tracked them for a few weeks—this isn't a medical diary, it's evidence.

- Include **when** symptoms happen: morning fog? Afternoon crash? Post-shower face-melt?

- Ask someone close to you to describe what they see when you're symptomatic. Preferably something more useful than "you look like a haunted duvet."

Make a "Greatest Hits of Me Not Coping" highlight reel even better. Think: *"On Monday, I tried to put peanut butter in the kettle. On Wednesday, I forgot my PIN and burst into tears in Lidl."*

Use Analogies That Hit Hard

GPs are humans with imaginations, and sometimes the best way to describe your weird symptoms is by going complete metaphor:

- "My legs feel like overcooked spaghetti trapped in jeans."

- "My brain is a loading screen that never gets past 2%."

- "I feel like I've been unplugged from the mains but someone forgot to switch me off."

The goal isn't to be poetic—it's to *stick in their minds.*

Mention the NICE Guidelines (Not Just to Sound Clever)

You don't have to recite them from memory like you're auditioning for "Britain's Got Bureaucracy"—**mention that you know** what's recommended for Long Covid.

Drop in:

"I saw that NICE defines ongoing symptomatic COVID-19 as lasting 4–12 weeks, and post-COVID syndrome as longer than 12. I'm at week 14, and I'm still struggling."

It signals: "Hey, I've done my homework, and I'm not here because I have a mild case of Monday."

This makes it harder for them to do the dreaded dismissive head-tilt.

Try to Stay Calm (LOL, But Actually)

Yes, you're tired. You're dizzy. You forgot your middle name yesterday. But **the calmer and clearer you are, the more likely you are to** be taken seriously. Is this fair? No. Is it reality? Sadly, yes.

- Write a cheat sheet to take with you.

- Bring a friend or ask to record the appointment (if your GP allows it—some do).

- If emotions sneak up on you mid-sentence (as they do), take a beat and breathe. Or sob theatrically and blame "inflammation of the emotions."

Don't Be Afraid to Ask for More

If your GP says, "It's probably just stress," smile serenely and say:

"Can you write that so I can show you the Long Covid clinic I'm being referred to?"

Because that's the next step—**ask for a referral to a Long-Term COVID clinic**. These clinics exist to investigate and support ongoing symptoms. If they say there isn't one nearby:

- Ask if a nearby hospital or integrated care system manages referrals.

- Suggest (gently or with righteous fire) that they check NHS pathways for Long Covid support.

- Or, if all else fails, **demand one be built immediately out of Lego and pure rage**. (It may not help, but it will feel good.)

- Ask your GP about Long COVID clinics. Bring a symptom diary. Mention PEM.

- Reference NICE guidelines. Show them you mean business—even if that business is held together with caffeine, cortisol, and sheer bloody-mindedness.

- Ask for investigations like ECGs, blood tests, and chest X-rays—not to prove you're sick but to rule out anything more sinister (and get you taken seriously). And remember, these tests are often like looking at a landscape through a telescope. You will see a lot, but might look in the wrong place. It doesn't mean you are healthy; they saw nothing today. You're feeling poorly, there is a reason, and no, it does not automatically mean it is in your head.

And if they dismiss you? Politely request another doctor. Or not-so-politely, depending on how many spoons you have that day.

The Long Covid Clinics: A Ray of Hope

There are specialist NHS Long COVID clinics. They offer multidisciplinary support: physios, OTs, psychologists, and fatigue specialists. They're not everywhere and have waitlists, but they exist. Find one: Search "NHS Long Covid clinic near me" or ask your GP for a referral. Be persistent: If your GP says they don't know about it, gently refer them to the NHS website. You can also tattoo it on your forearm.

There is also the unicorn of Long Covid Clinics – the long Covid Vocational Clinic, which can support you in your job. They can help you return to work, overcome bumps in the pathway to success and redefine yourself in this new world. They are pure gold.

> **Summary (Because - Brain Fog and this bit is important)**
> - Symptoms lasting 12+ weeks? Book the GP.
> - Be specific, use metaphors, and bring notes.
> - Mention NICE guidelines to show you've done your homework.
> - Stay calm—or as close as you can while falling apart.
> - Ask for a referral. If you're told no, push back kindly but firmly. Or start assembling Lego outside the surgery.

Remember: **You're not being dramatic. You're being persistent. There's a difference.**

Part One - Summary for the Foggy.

- You had COVID. You "recovered." But you're still sick. That's Long Covid.

- It's real, it's common, and it's not your fault.

- Symptoms = extreme fatigue, brain fog, breathlessness, palpitations, aches, weird gut stuff, anxiety, and more.

- It affects all kinds of people, not just the unfit or anxious.

- No, it's not just stress. Or burnout. Or laziness.

- Doctors and scientists are still figuring it out — it's messy but being taken seriously.

- Possible causes: immune freakouts, tiny clots, viral leftovers, nervous system issues.

- Vaccines didn't cause Long Covid. COVID did.

- Myths and judgment are common. Ignore them.

- If you're still unwell after 12 weeks, get checked — use notes, metaphors, and ask for a referral.

- Long Covid is exhausting, confusing, invisible — and you're not alone.

- Healing isn't linear. It's a wobbly, wild ride. You're doing your best. That's enough.

> *"They said 'rest and hydrate.' I've been horizontal for a year, and I pee every 20 minutes.*
> *WHERE'S MY CURE?"*

Part Two - WTF Do I Feel Like This?

Post Viral Syndrome or being dragged backwards, in slow motion, through a hedge.

Symptoms

It is hard to dig into the symptom list, as it is, frankly, terrifying. But this is an honest and brave book, and so are you.

Long-term COVID-19 is still being researched, and knowledge is expanding every day. Some of these symptoms will drop off the list in time, but we are all different, which might help you make sense of things. Remember, though, that not everything is Long-Term COVID-19, and if you are unsure, seek a medical opinion.

It's a lot. Just remember, you don't have to collect them all. Have a biscuit and breathe.

Fatigue – Am I Dying or Just Really, Really Tired?

Let's be clear: this isn't ordinary tiredness. This is industrial-strength fatigue. The tiredness that makes you need a nap after getting dressed. It makes you cry when you drop your spoon.

What's the Difference Between Tired and Long Covid Tired?

Normal tiredness: "I'm a bit sleepy; I stayed up watching Bake Off reruns. "Long Covid tired: "I blinked too hard and now must lie down. My bones are exhausted from holding me up "Sleep does not help long-term COVID fatigue. It's not laziness or lack of motivation. It's a systemic energy collapse.

Let's Talk About PEM

One of the crown jewels of Long Covid is Post-Exertional Malaise (PEM). This delightful feature means that if you do something even mildly active — a walk, a Zoom call, loading the dishwasher — you might pay for it with a crash that lasts hours or days. It's like your body sends you a passive-aggressive note saying: "That was cute. Don't do it again." Sound Familiar? You Might Be Crossing Over With POTS or ME/CFS

Many Long Covid sufferers show signs of conditions like:

- ME/CFS (Myalgic Encephalomyelitis / Chronic Fatigue Syndrome)

- POTS (Postural Orthostatic Tachycardia Syndrome)

Both are complex, poorly understood, and frustratingly underdiagnosed.

The overlaps include:

- Heart rate spikes when standing

- Dizziness

- Temperature sensitivity

- Digestive weirdness

Again, not all GPs are up to date on this. That's not a slight — they're overwhelmed and underfunded. But it means you might need to bring the science to the surgery.

Brain Fog - Damn, I Forgot What This Chapter Was About

B rain fog is the neurological cherry on top of the Long Covid sundae.

What It Feels Like

Forgetting names, faces, and tasks. Struggling to follow conversations. Losing your train of thought like it derailed at Clapham Junction. Mixing up words ("laundry banana" instead of "laundry basket")

Why It Happens

Studies are ongoing but may involve inflammation, lack of oxygen, or neurological damage. What we do know is that it's real, and it's not because you're getting old.

Coping Tips

Write everything down: Sticky notes, digital reminders, fridge magnets. Use timers and alarms: For meds, calls, even brushing your teeth. Break tasks into small chunks. Declutter your brain space: Try mindfulness or guided meditation (but skip the 45-minute YouTube ones with harps and dolphins)

Solidarity Corner

- One woman put her keys in the fridge and butter in her handbag.

- A man forgot his address while ordering a pizza.

- Another spent a week calling her cat "Steve". Her cat is named Biscuit.

- A woman who left the keys in the, very obviously open, front door and went shopping... (Hi!)

Humour helps. Acceptance helps more. Brain fog is frustrating, but it's not a character flaw. Be kind to yourself. You're doing great even without knowing what day it is.

Breathing/ Dizziness and the Body

The part where your body forgets how to be a body

One of the more dramatic (and frankly rude) features of Long Covid is the way your body randomly decides **oxygen is optional, standing is a thrill ride**, and your **heart thinks it's in a rave**. You walk up one flight of stairs, and your chest is pounding like you've just done a Tough Mudder in wellies. You turn your head too fast, and your living room does a fun little spin. You breathe… weird.

It's terrifying. It isn't very clear. And no, you're not making it up.

Let's break down this trifecta of "What fresh hell is this?": breathing weirdness, dizziness, and heart chaos.

The Breathing Bit (a.k.a. Am I Actually Out of Breath or Just Broken?)

Shortness of breath in Long Covid is common and deeply unsettling. It might hit you:

- Going upstairs (which now qualifies as Everest)

- Mid-sentence (fun!)

- While resting (double fun!)

But here's the thing: it's not about your lungs for many people. It's about **how your body regulates breath**, oxygen delivery, and panic. Even if your oxygen saturation is perfect (thank you, pulse oximeter obsession), you may still *feel* like you can't get air in. This is real. This is common. This is not "just in your head."

Some people develop **dysfunctional breathing patterns** post-Covid — like upper chest breathing, breath-holding, or over-breathing (hyperventilation). These don't appear on a chest X-ray, but your nervous system notices.

What Helps:
- **Breathing retraining** (via a physio or guided videos)

- **Paced breathing**: Try 4 seconds in, 6 seconds out

- **Box breathing**: In-4, hold-4, out-4, hold-4 — but only if that feels okay

- **Diaphragmatic breathing** (a.k.a. belly breathing — because nothing's ever easy with Long Covid, not even breathing)

Also, lying down and crying because it's all a bit much is *also valid*.

The Dizziness Bit (a.k.a. "I Got Up Too Fast and Now I Live on the Floor")

Let's talk about **dysautonomia**. That's the fancy word: "your automatic systems — like heart rate, blood pressure, temperature control, digestion — have all gone rogue."

You might be dealing with:

- **Light-headedness** when standing

- **Black spots** in vision

- **Feeling like you're floating or swaying**

- **"Drunk without the fun" wobbliness**

- **Vertigo**, spinning rooms, or sudden "woosh" sensations

This is because your **autonomic nervous system** is acting like someone unplugged it and plugged it back incorrectly.

One common culprit? **Postural Orthostatic Tachycardia Syndrome** (POTS) — a condition where your heart rate spikes abnormally just from standing up.

POTS and other forms of orthostatic intolerance are being reported more and more in Long Covid cases. And no, Brenda, it's not "just dehydration."

The Heart Bit (a.k.a. "Why Is My Chest Thumping Like There's a Drum Rave Inside Me?")

Let's not sugarcoat it — **Long Covid does weird things to your heart.**

You might notice:

- **Palpitations** (thudding, fluttering, racing)

- **Tachycardia** (heart rate over 100 bpm at rest or on standing)
- **Chest discomfort**
- **Skipped beats**
- **Feeling like your heart forgot how to beat**

It feels scary, and it should always be checked out. But for many, heart tests come back "normal." (Which is a strange kind of gaslighting your body does to itself.)

This doesn't mean nothing's wrong. It means:

- Your heart muscle *might* be fine...

- ...but your **nervous system is sending the wrong signals**

In other words: you're not imagining it. You're not "just anxious." Your body is having a full-blown communication breakdown.

So What Do We Do?

This is not a "just breathe and stay positive" situation. It's a "support your nervous system and ask for help while lying down with snacks" situation.

First: Get Checked

- Ask for an **ECG**, blood pressure lying/standing, and blood tests

- Mention **POTS, orthostatic intolerance**, and **autonomic dysfunction**

- Request a **referral to cardiology or a Long Covid clinic**

If you're told "it's just anxiety," smile sweetly and ask them to put that in writing — so you can take it to someone who understands your symptoms.

Practical Things That Might Help
- **Increase salt and fluids** (if safe for you): Helps blood volume, which can stabilise symptoms

- **Compression garments** (hello, sexy flight socks): Support circulation

- **Slow position changes**: Sit up, wait, stand up, wait, then move like a majestic tortoise

- **Breathing exercises** (see earlier — yes, again)

- **Cooling down**: Heat can make symptoms worse

- **Heart rate tracking**: Some find wearable devices helpful for pacing

Also helpful is **not panicking** every time your heart gets excited about you loading the dishwasher. Easier said than done. But still true.

> **Recap for the Foggy**
> - Breathing feels weird? It's common. Try slow, belly breathing.
>
> - Dizzy when standing? Could be POTS or autonomic weirdness.
>
> - Heart doing the cha-cha? Get it checked — but it might

be dysfunction, not damage.

- This is scary, but it's real. And you're not the only one.

Your Friend On the Sofa

Your body is not broken — it's *recalibrating*. Slowly. Grumpily. And not on your preferred schedule.

So if you feel like a winded gazelle after getting the post, or your heart races when you change your socks, you are not alone. You're just living in the haunted house of Long Covid physiology, where everything beeps, wobbles, and panics for no good reason.

Go gently. Go slowly. Sit down a lot. Drink water. Breathe like you mean it. And if all else fails, lie on the floor and whisper, "This is fine" until your heart gets bored and behaves.

You're doing better than you think.

THE BRAIN, THE MOOD, AND THE JUDDERING MESS

Let's talk brains. And nerves. And moods. And why do you suddenly feel like a jittery 2003 PC trying to run ten tabs and Microsoft Paint simultaneously?

Because here's the thing: **Long Covid doesn't just mess with your lungs and limbs — it breaks into your brain**, rearranges the furniture, deletes your emotional regulation files, and installs a flickering neon sign that reads *"System error: please try again later."*

This chapter is about what happens when your nervous system stops being polite and gets glitchy.

Anxiety, Depression & Emotional Mayhem – *No, you're not "just stressed."*

But stress, anxiety, and depression? Yes — they often tag along for the ride. Whether it's caused by neurological changes, trauma, isolation, or your body constantly sending "danger!" signals when you're trying to do your laundry, **your mental health can take a hit**.

What it might feel like:

- Waking with dread for no reason

- Crying at that one dog food advert with the sad piano music

- Feeling like you're floating *outside* of yourself

- Sudden spikes of terror (why? unknown!)

- Apathy and hopelessness, you can't "snap out of it"

- Needing 4 hours to psych yourself up for a 2-minute phone call

Some people report full-on **emotional detachment**. Others swing between "deep despair" and "intense rage because the dishwasher beeped too loudly."

It's not a character flaw. It's **neurological fallout**. The brain has *extreme* opinions about being inflamed and exhausted, and one of them is: "Let's feel absolutely everything. Or nothing. All at once."

Tremors, Judders, and Internal Vibrations *Or: Why do I Feel Like a Low-Budget Ghost is electrocuting me?*

Let's get to the truly unnerving stuff — the **tremors, twitching, judders**, and weird internal buzzing that makes you question whether you're being haunted or just poorly coded.

These symptoms are often underreported, under researched, and wildly misunderstood.

They might show up as:
- Hands or limbs shaking uncontrollably (sometimes only at rest, sometimes during movement)

- Whole-body judders or spasms, especially when trying to sleep

- A strange, **internal vibrating** sensation — like your bones are buzzing, but no one can see it

- Eye twitches, lip trembles, jaw clenching

- Sudden jerks (myoclonic movements) — like your body just jumped at nothing

And here's the kicker: your tests? It might come back to normal, which makes you feel like maybe you *are* just possessed. (You're not.)

Doctors are starting to recognise this as part of the **neurological aftermath** of Long Covid — likely tied to autonomic dysfunction, brain inflammation, or small fibre nerve irritation. It's a **nervous system hiccup** that feels like your body's running static through the wiring.

Some describe it as feeling "like a phone on vibrate... inside my chest." Others call it "buzzing bones" or "popcorn legs." It's bizarre. It's real. And you're not imagining it.

Other Fun Neurological Oddities:
- **Light and sound sensitivity** – because being tired isn't enough, now lightbulbs hurt

- **Tinnitus** – persistent ringing, whooshing, or buzzing in your ears

- **Balance problems** – walking into doorframes for no reason

- **Visual disturbances** – blurry vision, floaters, trouble focusing

- **Sensory overload** – sounds feel like they're stabbing you; supermarket lighting makes you cry

- **Dissociation** – like watching your life from 6 inches outside your body

What Might Actually Help?

(Disclaimer: Nothing fixes this entirely, but some things may calm the chaos.)

- **Pacing**. Your brain needs rest, too — mental exertion can crash you like physical exertion.

- **Reducing stimulation**. Low light, noise-cancelling headphones, and blue light filters. Your senses need a break.

- **Gentle grounding techniques** – 5-4-3-2-1 (5 things you see, 4 feel, 3 hear, etc.). Or pet a cat. Works for me.

- **Journaling or voice notes** – to track patterns (and remember why you walked into the kitchen).

- **Therapy** (if accessible) – especially trauma-informed or neuro-aware therapists

- **Medication** – some people find help with SSRIs, anti-anxiety meds, low-dose naltrexone, or meds targeting nerve pain (talk to a GP who believes in actual medicine)

And sometimes? **Just knowing it's real** helps.

Recap for the Foggy:

- Brain fog = cognitive dysfunction. Not your fault. Not forever.

- Anxiety & depression are **part of the illness**, not your personality failing.

- Tremors, internal buzzing, jerks = common neurological symptoms. Often terrifying, rarely dangerous.

- You're not haunted. But your nervous system *is* on the fritz.

- You're not alone. You're not broken. You're just living in hard mode.

Your Friend on the Sofa

Long Covid isn't just a physical illness — it's a **whole-body, whole-mind experience** that messes with your nervous system like it's trying to remix your personality. Some days you'll feel like a haunted house—other days, like a sentient potato with WiFi glitches.

But through the fear, the fog, and the frustrating lack of understanding from others, remember this: **you are still in there.**

> Shaky, buzzing, overwhelmed, maybe — but not gone. Not crazy. Not broken. Not imagining it. You are surviving a neurological storm. And somehow, still managing to put on socks (or at least *try*).
>
> And that's bloody impressive.

THE MUSCLES, THE JOINTS, AND THE BETRAYAL

L et's get one thing out of the way: you're not imagining this pain.
If you've found yourself waking up feeling like you've been folded into an origami crane overnight... or that your limbs are stuffed with sandbags and resentment... or that your neck, back, and shoulders are locked in a full-scale mutiny — congratulations, you've unlocked the **musculoskeletal bonus level** of Long Covid.

It's achy. It isn't very clear. It's exhausting. And yes — it's real.

So What's Going On?
Long Covid can affect muscles, joints, fascia (that stretchy webby stuff), tendons, and all the little connective tissues you **never knew existed** until they started screaming at you whenever you got out of a chair.

Some people experience **new pain**, some have **old injuries resurface**, and some feel like they've just been lightly beaten with baguettes every time they try to stand up. For many, the pain **moves around**, appears randomly, and refuses to behave.

This is not a fun mystery. It is the **"Why do I feel like I pulled a hamstring brushing my teeth?"** kind.

Common Musculoskeletal Symptoms in Long Covid:

- **Muscle pain** (anywhere, everywhere, all at once)

- **Joint stiffness** (especially in the morning or after resting)

- **Cramping or spasms** (sudden and rude)

- **Muscle weakness** (limbs feel floppy, shaky, or jelly-like)

- **Delayed-onset pain** (you feel fine *during* the walk... and then collapse six hours later)

- **Burning sensations in muscles** (hello nerve involvement!)

- **Back pain, shoulder pain, neck pain** — even in places that were fine before

- **"Heavy limbs"** — like gravity just doubled, but only in your legs

- **Fascial tightness** — that skin-stretching, body-wrapping tension that makes you feel shrink-wrapped

All this, without ever running a marathon. Unless you count *standing to unload the dishwasher* as a marathon, which, in fairness, it now is.

What Does the Pain *Feel* Like?

People describe it in a thousand creatively miserable ways. Some highlights:

- "Like I've been hit with a sack of potatoes in the night."

- "Like my bones are too heavy for my body."

- "Like my muscles were filled with acid and left to marinate."

- "Like I aged 50 years overnight and forgot how joints are supposed to move."

Pain may be **burning, throbbing, aching, stabbing**, or **a dull, full-body grumble**. It might stay in one place or tour your body like a moody backpacker. One day, it's your knees. Next, your hands. Then your shoulder blade for no good reason.

Exertion can make it worse. Thanks, Post-Exercise Malaise **(PEM)**. Nothing says "I love consequences" like doing gentle yoga and needing to lie down for 48 hours.

Why Does This Happen?

Doctors are still figuring it out (of course), but possible culprits include:

- **Inflammation** – Your immune system is throwing an endless tantrum

- **Nerve involvement** – Small fibre neuropathy may cause pain, burning, and twitching

- **Autonomic dysfunction** – Messes with blood flow to muscles, causing that "heavy legs" or "dead arm" feeling

- **Mitochondrial fatigue** – Your cells are tired. Really tired. Like, "ran out of petrol halfway through brushing your hair," tired

- **Deconditioning** – Not the whole story, but being bed-bound or limited for weeks/months *does* reduce muscle strength and joint flexibility

- **Myofascial tension** – The body's connective tissue gets tense and sticky, like cling film you can't peel off

So What Can You Actually *Do* About It?

Here's the unglamorous truth: there's no magic fix. But some things can **manage the pain**, support recovery, and help you feel more human.

Things That Might Help:
- **Pacing.** (Yes, again. Sorry.) Rest before you crash. Not after.

- **Heat or ice.** Microwaveable wheat bags and hot baths = heroes.

- **Stretching gently.** Very gently. Think "cat yawning," not "Instagram yoga."

- **Pain relief.** If you need over-the-counter meds, muscle rubs, and other products, talk to your GP about prescriptions.

- **Physiotherapy.** *But only from someone who understands Long Covid.* Aggressive rehab can backfire.

- **Massage therapy.** Light touch, myofascial release, or lymphatic drainage — not sports massage unless you're into weeping.

- **Magnesium supplements or sprays.** Sometimes it helps with cramps and spasms.

- **Mobility aids.** Walking sticks, grabbers, chairs in the shower — all rock 'n' roll.

Avoid:

- "Just push through the pain." This isn't a gym slogan. It's a crash waiting to happen.

- "You just need to get moving again." Tell that to your calves, which are made of cement and spite.

- "Stretch more." More isn't always better if your fascia is inflamed or your nerves are irritated.

- Taking more pain killers than allowed. Be very careful, particularly with paracetamol.

The Bare Minimum for Bad Pain Days:

- Don't move more than you have to

- Rest in supportive positions (pillows everywhere — under knees, behind neck, under arms)

- Drink water (even if it feels useless)

- Apply heat, take the meds, breathe slowly

- Don't guilt yourself for not "exercising through it"

This is a **recovery**, not a boot camp.

> **Your Friend on the Sofa**
>
> Pain is invisible, which means other people don't see it or understand it and often say things like, "You just need to stretch more!" or "Have you tried Pilates?" or "Oh yeah, I get tired too."
>
> Feel free to ignore them while lying flat, wrapped in heat packs and radiating sarcasm.
>
> This isn't in your head. It's in your joints, your muscles, your fascia, and your bones — and it's exhausting. But it's not a moral failing. It doesn't mean you're broken. It means your body is fighting a long, weird battle — and you're doing your absolute best with a meat suit that keeps glitching.
>
> So go slow. Sit often. Swear freely. And if all you managed today was a slow shuffle to the kettle with pain in places you didn't know you had, that's a win.

GUT FEELINGS

Welcome to the glamorous world of **gastric symptoms in Long Covid**, where your digestion has completely lost the plot, your food preferences have regressed to "toast or death," and your stomach behaves like it's starring in a melodrama.

Let's get one thing straight: **you're not being fussy**. This isn't about being picky, anxious, or "sensitive." It's about your once perfectly functional digestive system now throwing daily tantrums over things like yoghurt, onions, or *air*.

This is your body's internal monologue now:

"You want me to eat *what*? At this time of day? Without lying down for three hours first? HOW DARE YOU."

So What's Actually Happening?

Many people with Long Covid experience **gastrointestinal (GI) symptoms**, even without stomach issues during the initial infection.

For some, it starts **during** COVID and never quite resolves. For others, it creeps in weeks or months later like an unwanted houseguest who won't stop rearranging your internal organs.

These symptoms can be:
- Mild but annoying

- Horrific and life-altering

- Or, more often, both, and highly unpredictable

Common Gastric Symptoms in Long Covid
- **Nausea** – constant, random, or specifically triggered by movement/smell/stress/food/the existence of food

- **Diarrhoea** – sudden, urgent, explosive (a crowd favourite!)

- **Constipation** – equally glamorous

- **Bloating** – the "is she pregnant or just possessed by bread?" kind

- **Acid reflux/heartburn** – spicy regrets at 3 a.m.

- **Burping, gassiness, flatulence** – let's not pretend we're not making our own soundtracks at this point

- **Stomach pain or cramps** – sometimes dull, sometimes stabby, always confusing

- **Food intolerances or sensitivities** – things you used to eat? Now betrayals.

- **Loss of appetite or early fullness** – you try, and your gut goes "Nah."

- **Weight loss or gain** – the chaotic seesaw of unpredictable eating and absorption

Your gut has joined your nervous system in the "We Quit" union.

What Might Be Going On?
Let's throw some science at it, shall we?
Possible causes include:

- **Vagal nerve dysfunction** – the vagus nerve runs from the brain to the gut. Covid might irritate it, and your stomach goes rogue.

- **Autonomic dysfunction** – also affects digestion (surprise! Your body forgot how to multitask).

- **Mast cell activation**—Some people develop overactive immune cells, which can trigger reactions to foods, smells, and chemicals.

- **Post-viral IBS** – Covid, like many viruses, may trigger long-term digestive chaos.

- **Gastroparesis** (in some cases) – delayed stomach emptying, which makes food hang around like a bad decision.

- **Microbiome disruption** – your gut bacteria? Also tired.

Of course, doctors may run tests and say, "Everything's normal." It is like hearing your house is structurally sound while on fire.

What Might Actually Help (Sometimes)

There's no one-size-fits-all approach, but here are some strategies people have found helpful:

For Nausea:
- Ginger (tea, capsules, chews)
- Peppermint (tea, oil — *not* to be confused with essential oil shots, which: no)
- Small, frequent meals
- Dry, bland foods (crackers, toast, beige joy)
- Anti-nausea meds from your GP (you deserve them!)

For Reflux:
- Smaller meals, no eating late at night
- Raise the head of your bed (or stack pillows until you're basically upright)
- Avoid trigger foods (sorry, tomato sauce)
- Ask your GP about PPIs or H2 blockers if it's severe

For Bloating and Gas:
- Low FODMAP diet (short-term, supervised ideally — not a forever thing)
- Peppermint capsules
- Gentle movement (if possible), abdominal massage
- Probiotics (some find relief, others just more farts)

For Constipation:
- Fibre — but introduce slowly unless you enjoy abdominal Morse code
- Water (obviously)
- Gentle laxatives (GP-approved, not your nan's prune juice prescription)
- Magnesium citrate (bonus: may help with sleep and cramps)

For Diarrhoea:
- Stick to low-fibre, gentle foods during flares
- Rehydration salts or electrolyte drinks
- Ask about bile acid malabsorption (a sneaky post-viral issue)

Eating with a Moody Gut: Survival Tips
- **Keep it simple.** Think: toast, rice, bananas, broth, chicken, soft veg
- **Avoid high-fat, rich meals** (your gut is not currently interested in feasting)
- **Don't force it** — eat what you can, when you can, in small amounts
- **Track triggers** if you have the brain space (a food diary, or "the notebook of doom")
- **Eat sitting up, chew slowly, stay upright after** — treat eating like a science experiment

Also, if your body only wants beige, don't feel guilty. You can reintroduce colour and nutrients when your body is ready. Survival is the first priority. *Kale can wait.*

When to Speak to a Doctor

Yes, gastric symptoms are common — but that doesn't mean you should suffer in silence. See your GP if:

- You're losing weight unintentionally
- You can't eat without feeling awful
- You've got ongoing diarrhoea, blood in stool, or severe pain
- You feel full after a few bites, or food seems to sit in your stomach forever
- You're struggling to stay hydrated

And if your GP says, "It's just anxiety", kindly ask them to explain how anxiety gives you explosive diarrhoea every time you eat a peach.

Foggy Recap

- Your gut is not okay, and you're not imagining it.
- Nausea, bloating, reflux, cramps, diarrhoea, and food reactions are all part of the Long Covid buffet.
- Some things can help, but it's trial-and-error, **not failure if something doesn't work.**
- You deserve to eat, be comfortable, and *not live in fear of soup.*

> **Your Friend on the Sofa**
> Living with a malfunctioning digestive system is **miserable, embarrassing**, and **utterly exhausting**. You're managing symptoms that are invisible, unpredictable, and often not taken seriously — all while trying to eat enough to stay upright.

THE WEIRD AND THE WIDESPREAD

Long Covid is the gift that keeps on giving — like a terrible subscription box filled with mystery symptoms, missing instruction manuals, and a note that says *"Good luck!"*

By now, you've probably heard about the usual suspects: fatigue, breathlessness, and brain fog. But let's talk about the **supporting cast** — the lesser-known, still-exhausting, and often wildly inconvenient symptoms that make you wonder if your body is trying out for a medical drama.

Yes, these are real. Yes, other people have them too. And no, you're not being *dramatic*. You're being *systemically dismantled at a cellular level*.

Let's dive in.

Circulatory / Autonomic Shenanigans
(Your body's autopilot has left the building.)

- **POTS (Postural Orthostatic Tachycardia Syndrome)**

  - The moment you stand up, your heart rate does parkour. You feel faint, shaky, and ready to collapse just from brushing your hair. Standing still is now an extreme sport.

- **Cold Extremities**

  - Toes like ice cubes, fingers like tiny corpses. You could be wrapped in three blankets, and your feet are still auditioning for *Frozen 3*.

- **Flushing or Sweating Abnormalities**

  - Sometimes you're a furnace. Other times, you're freezing. Sometimes you're sweating while cold, which feels like your body is trying to defy physics out of spite.

- **Low or Unstable Blood Pressure**

  - Feeling faint? Dizzy? Vision going spotty? Congratulations — your blood pressure is on its own personal rollercoaster and didn't invite you to the meeting.

Immune & Inflammatory Drama

Your immune system didn't get the "stop attacking" memo.

- **Swollen Lymph Nodes**

  - Neck lumpy? Armpits tender? Feeling like you're "about to come down with something" for eight months straight? That's just your lymph system, sighing loudly.

- **Low-Grade Fevers or Chills**
    - You don't have a temperature... except when you do. You're cold in July and clammy in December. It's like your body's trying to gaslight your thermostat.

- **Reactivation of Old Viruses**
    - Shingles, EBV (mono), cold sores — old viruses love making comebacks in Long Covid. It's like your immune system said, "Let's bring the gang back together!"

Ear, Nose & Throat (ENT) Chaos
(You know, just in case you wanted to stop enjoying food and hearing correctly)

- **Loss or Distortion of Smell (Anosmia / Parosmia)**
    - Everything smells like burnt onions, petrol, or sewage — even when it shouldn't. You miss the simple joy of a cup of coffee that doesn't smell like death.

- **Loss or Distortion of Taste**
    - Spicy things taste metallic. Sweet things taste sour. Or maybe everything tastes like nothing. Either way, your tongue has officially resigned.

- **Sore Throat**
    - Persistent, nagging, therefor-no-reason kind of sore. Not strep. Not flu. Just... there. Being annoying.

- **Ear Pain or Pressure**

○ Crackling ears, blocked ears, sharp pain — like someone shoved a balloon animal in your ear canal. Fun!

Dental / Oral Nightmares
(Your teeth and gums got the virus memo, too.)
- **Mouth Ulcers**

Painful, recurring, and always arriving when you *don't* have Bonjela nearby.

- **Gum Issues or Sensitivity**

Bleeding, puffiness, sensitivity — even if your dentist says your oral hygiene is "perfect." (Thanks, immune dysregulation!)

- **Tooth Pain (Unexplained)**

Random zings of pain in random teeth. Sometimes it feels like your entire jaw is sulking. No cavity. No cause. Just vibes.

Skin & Hair Mayhem
(Because your body just had to add drama to your scalp.)
- **Hair Loss (Telogen Effluvium)**

  ○ Clumps in the shower, strands on the pillow, a tiny panic every time you touch your scalp. It's temporary (usually), but distressing.

- **Rashes**

  ○ Itchy, hives, eczema-like, or red and blotchy. Sometimes looks like sunburn, sometimes looks like stress. Always looks like *why*?

- **Skin Sensitivity or Burning**

    ○ Your skin hurts to touch. Even clothes feel "too much." You're suddenly starring in your slow-motion lava commercial.

- **Mental Health & Sensory Overload**

It's not "just stress" — but wow, stress is now also a full-body experience

- **Panic Attacks**

    ○ Out of the blue, body-wide fear, pounding heart, shaking hands — usually for no identifiable reason. Because you needed *more* adrenaline.

- **Emotional Dysregulation**

    ○ Crying over supermarket lighting. Rage because someone sneezed too loudly. Feeling like you're 12 moods in one hour. You're not unstable — your brain is just inflamed and overstimulated.

- **Intrusive Thoughts**

    ○ Sudden, unwanted thoughts—dark, strange, or unsettling—are common, distressing, and often temporary. They are worth mentioning to someone supportive.

- **Sensory Overload**

    ○ Sound is too loud, light is too bright, and textures feel unbearable. Crowds? Absolutely not. Your nervous system is on high alert, and *everyone* is too much.

> **Quick Foggy Recap**
> - **Autonomic weirdness** = dizziness, cold hands, heart rate chaos, unpredictable blood pressure
>
> - **Immune chaos** = swollen glands, fevers, viral reactivations
>
> - **ENT drama** = loss of smell/taste, sore throat, ear pressure
>
> - **Dental surprises** = ulcers, gum pain, tooth zaps
>
> - **Skin & hair** = hair loss, rashes, nerve zings
>
> - **Mental health & sensory overload** = panic, rage, emotional WTFs, and light/sound meltdowns

> **Your Friend on the Sofa**
>
> Long Covid isn't just a lung issue. It's a **full-body system rebellion**, and these lesser-known symptoms deserve just as much attention and compassion as the "big" ones.
>
> So if your hair is falling out, your toes are freezing, your gums hurt, and you're crying over a cheese advert — you are not broken. You are just navigating a complex, multi-system condition while the world expects you to "just get on with it."

Go easy. Track what you can. Ask for help where you need it. And **remember: You're not a hypochondriac. You're just very, very observant about your slowly unravelling body.**

And that? It's survival in style.

Part Two - Summary for the Foggy

- **Fatigue**: Not tired. **System shutdown.** Getting dressed = a full day's work.

- **Brain Fog**: Forgot your cat's name? Normal. Thought "banana" meant laundry basket? Also normal.

- **Breathing/Dizzy/Heart**: Your body thinks air is optional, standing is skydiving, and your heart's in a rave.

- **Muscles & Joints**: Pain for no reason. Like you were beaten up by your own duvet.

- **Twitching/Vibrating**: Internal earthquake. You buzz, you spasm, no one else can see it.

- **Gut Drama**: Everything you eat is now a dare. Toast = friend. Everything else = betrayal.

- **Bonus Weirdness**: Cold toes, zingy teeth, light hurts, and you cried over a spoon.

- **Recap**: You're not lazy, crazy, or dramatic. Just running Long Covid on hard mode.

"I asked if I'd ever feel normal again.

    The doctor said, 'Define normal.'

    I said, 'You know — like pre-COVID... when I still had a career, a waistline, and hopes.'"

Part Three - HTF Do I Live Now?

Living Life in Low Power Mode

Let's face it: daily life with Long Covid can feel like trying to run a marathon with flip-flops, a cold, and no sense of direction. When your energy is limited, and your body plays by its own chaotic rules, even the most basic tasks—like brushing your teeth or opening the curtains—can become epic quests.

This chapter is your practical, no-nonsense, slightly sarcastic guide to surviving the mundane realities of living with Long Covid. Think of it as the IKEA instructions for pacing life: confusing at first but ultimately helpful.

Spoonie Economics: Budgeting Energy Like It's Gold

You may have heard of the Spoon Theory. If not, here's the short version: imagine your energy each day as a limited number of spoons.

Every activity costs a spoon (or five), and when you run out, you're done. No credit. No overdraft. Just crash.

Welcome to Spoonie Economics. It's about budgeting your energy like you're living off coupons in a cost-of-living crisis.

Daily Energy Audit:
- Write down your daily tasks.
- Estimate the cost of each spoon.
- Prioritise like your life depends on it (because some days, it does).

High-Spoon Tasks (use with caution):
- Showering
- Cooking from scratch
- Vacuuming
- Anything involving stairs

Low-Spoon Wins:
- Sitting outside for 10 minutes
- Reheating food
- Using dry shampoo
- Accepting help

Top Tip: Always reserve a few spoons. Think of them as your emergency chocolate stash—for surprise crashes, toddler tantrums, or spontaneous emotional spirals.

SHOWERING WITHOUT WEEPING

Yes, it's just water. No, it's not simple. Showering with Long Covid can feel like climbing Kilimanjaro in a wetsuit.

How to Bathe in Survival Mode:

1. **Sit Down.** Get a shower stool or chair. No shame. Sitting uses fewer spoons.

2. **Switch to Evening Showers.** Mornings are for waking up and surviving, while evening showers allow you to collapse into bed straight after.

3. **Shower Wipes are Valid.** Wipe baths? Totally acceptable. Clean is clean.

4. **Dry Shampoo & Deodorant = Winning.** You're not grimy, you're conserving resources.

5. **Skip the Hair.** Washing hair = a multi-spoon event. Only do it when necessary, or enlist help.

Energy-Saving Bathroom Tips
- Use a robe to dry yourself slowly.
- Prep clothes and towels ahead of time.
- Keep the bathroom ventilated to avoid overheating.

COOKING WHEN YOUR ARMS FEEL LIKE LEAD

When you're ill, food prep needs to be fast and easy and not involve the word "julienne."

Spoonie Cooking Rules:

1. **Batch Cook on Good Days.** Use energy when you have it to prep freezer meals.

2. **Pre-Chopped is Your Friend.** Frozen veg? Yes. Pre-cut fruit? Absolutely.

3. **One-Pot Wonders.** Less washing up, less effort.

4. **Air Fryers/Microwaves > Ovens.** Time + energy saved = worth it.

5. **Meal Prep Zones.** Sit at the counter to chop. Use perching stools.

Spoon-Friendly Meals:
- Pre-made soup with toast
- Eggs in any form
- Wraps (with whatever's in the fridge)
- Smoothies (if tolerated)
- Instant noodles with added veg

Pro Tip: Use paper plates on flare days. No washing up, no shame.

CLEANING WITHOUT COLLAPSING

The dust can wait. Your health can't. But here are some hacks to help maintain a vaguely hygienic environment without ending up horizontal.

Cleaning in Crisis Mode:

1. **Micro-Cleaning:** 5-minute tasks only. Set a timer. Stop when it buzzes.

2. **Clean from a Chair:** Wipe surfaces while seated. Bring the mess to you.

3. **Use Tools:** Lightweight vacuum? Long-handled dusters? Robot mop? Yes, yes, yes.

4. **Declutter Your Space (Slowly):** Less stuff = less to clean.

5. **Prioritise Zones:** Kitchen, loo, bed. The rest is a bonus.

Smart Hacks:
- Use antibacterial wipes for quick fixes.
- Keep cleaning supplies in multiple rooms.
- Ask for help. Delegate. Bribe with snacks if needed.

Managing Family Life When You Feel Like a Ghost

Whether you're a parent, partner, or both, Long COVID doesn't put a pause on family responsibilities. But it does mean playing life on hard mode.

Communicate Like a Legend:
- Explain energy limits using spoon analogies.
- Create a code for "I'm about to crash" (e.g. waving a tea towel).
- Share a calendar to mark flare days or appointments.

Get the Kids Involved:
- Age-appropriate chores can be empowering.
- Make tidying a game (yes, you can bribe with screen time).
- Use visual schedules or timers for routines.

Partner Protocols:
- Share a weekly energy check-in.
- Be honest about needs.
- Schedule in rest time like appointments.

Family Hacks:
- Lazy dinners = bonding dinners (picnic in the living room!)
- Quiet play is golden. Invest in puzzles, audiobooks, and LEGO.
- Don't feel bad about screen time. It's a survival tool.

GOOD DAY / BAD DAY ROUTINES

Let's break down what a realistic day might look like in two flavours: Good and Bad.

Sample Good Day:
Morning:
- Wake slowly with water and meds
- Gentle stretches in bed
- Toast + tea breakfast
- Short seated shower
- 1 hour of activity (admin, calls, emails)

Afternoon:
- Lunch (leftovers)

- 1-hour rest/nap
- Light activity (folding laundry seated)
- 15-minute fresh air break

Evening:
- Easy dinner (helped or ordered)
- Watch TV with feet up
- Early bed with audiobook or meditation app

Sample Bad Day:
Morning:
- Wake up feeling like you never slept
- Skip shower, use wipes and dry shampoo
- Toast, if possible. Tea, definitely.
- Stay in bed or on the sofa with a heat pack

Afternoon:
- Cereal for lunch
- Nap or mindless TV
- Track symptoms if able
- Accept help without guilt

Evening:
- Eat what's available

- Avoid bright lights and noise
- Bed early, no pressure

> **Your Friend on the Sofa**
>
> Living with Long COVID demands creativity, compassion, and a deep respect for one's body's limits. These hacks aren't just survival tools; they're acts of rebellion against a world that values productivity over well-being.
>
> You are not lazy. You are adapting. You are not failing. You are surviving.
>
> Go slow. Be kind to yourself. And if all you did today was read this chapter in bed with crumbs on your chest, that counts.
>
> Big spoons to you.

Part Three - Summary for the Foggy.

- **Spoons = Currency**: Budget energy like you're broke and every task is expensive. Save some for emergencies (or toddler tantrums)

- **Showering is an Extreme Sport**: Sit down, switch to evening showers, and embrace dry shampoo. Clean is clean—even with wipes.

- **Cooking= Minimal Effort Meals**: Batch-cook on good days, love your microwave, and never feel bad about instant noodles or paper plates.

- **Cleaning? Barely.**: 5-minute bursts, sit while wiping stuff, and use gadgets. Prioritise bathroom, kitchen, bed. The dust elsewhere can wait.

- **Family Life on Hard Mode**: Communicate limits clearly,

let kids help, share energy check-ins with partners, and make quiet play sacred.

- **Good Day vs. Bad Day**: Plan flexible routines. Good days = light activity with rests. Bad days = survival mode (tea, toast, TV, bed).

- Final Thought: You're not lazy—you're adapting. Go slow, be kind to yourself, and if all you managed today was reading this in bed… it count

> *"It's called Long COVID because 'eternal suffering with no refund' didn't test well in focus groups."*

Part Four - WTF Happened To Me?

The Stranger In the Mirror

Chronic illness has many charming calling cards: fatigue, brain fog, mysterious aches, and a sudden tendency to cry at supermarket adverts. But perhaps the most disorienting gift it bestows is the total upheaval of your self-image. One day, you're bustling around like the dependable human kettle you once were; the next, you're bloated, wrinkled, and staring into the mirror thinking, *"Who the hell is that tired-looking ghost impersonating me?"*

Long COVID has a knack for turning your body into a stranger—a creaky, unreliable, occasionally swollen stranger who steals your socks and naps without warning. And somewhere in that transformation, your confidence packs a small suitcase and checks out without so much as a goodbye note.

What Happened to My Face?

You may have noticed it in a photo. The first one you saw after the diagnosis – a picture taken at a birthday or a socially distanced barbecue, where you're smiling but your eyes look like they've seen the apocalypse. The face you remember – energised, sparkly, vaguely symmetrical – is gone. In its place: dark circles, slack skin, and a look that says, *"I've been awake since William the Conqueror popped over to Hastings for kebab."*

It's not vanity. Its identity. We all want to feel like ourselves. But illness doesn't care about your skincare routine or your 10,000 steps. It unpacks its bags, lounges on your collagen, and begins a slow but steady campaign to make you feel alien in your skin.

The Betrayal of the Body

Perhaps the cruellest part of chronic illness is how thoroughly your body stops playing for your team. The legs that used to dance, jog, or even reliably carry you to the loo now mutter *"meh"* at the first sign of movement. Your stamina? Evaporated. Your posture? Hunched like a guilty goblin. Your sense of ownership over your limbs? Fractured, at best.

You used to *trust* your body. It wasn't perfect, but it was familiar. Now, every creak and twinge feels like a coded message in a language you've forgotten. The result? A kind of existential homesickness. Not just for your old life but for the body that lets you live it without issuing hourly threat-level warnings.

The Weight of It All

Let's address the elephant in the room – the fluctuating elephant on the bathroom scales.

Chronic illness can send your weight into chaos. Maybe you've lost it because food became unappealing or exhausting. Perhaps you've gained because your mobility tanked and your diet consists mainly of toast and shame. Either way, your clothes don't fit, your joints are protesting, and your reflection feels like someone else's experiment.

And the worst part? The commentary – internal or otherwise. *"You'd feel better if you just lost some weight." "Maybe you're tired because you're inactive."* As though chronic illness were some motivational failure rather than an actual physiological ordeal. Spoiler: it's not your fault.

Identity Theft: The Confidence Heist

What no one tells you is that chronic illness doesn't just rob you of health – it **steals your confidence**. You used to stride. Now you shuffle. You used to say yes. Now you weigh every invitation like it's an Olympic event. You once stood in queues, carried bags, walked the dog – all without second-guessing your body's survival ability.

That confident person hasn't disappeared. They're just buried under a pile of symptom diaries, heating pads, and sheer exhaustion.

Rebuilding Trust with Your Body

It's tempting to see your body as the enemy. Treat it like a moody flatmate who's stopped doing the dishes and now only speaks in grunts and passive aggression. But here's the thing: this body, this cranky, battered, barely functioning meat suit, is still yours. And it's trying.

The goal isn't to return to the old you. That's unrealistic (and frankly, she wasn't that well-rested either). The goal is to **make peace**. To rebuild a relationship with your body based on realism, compassion, and low expectations.

Here's what that might look like:

- **Dress for comfort and joy.** Your body has changed, and so should your wardrobe. Nothing builds resentment like a waistband that cuts off circulation and hope.

- **Celebrate small wins.** Managed a shower? A walk around the block? Didn't cry during breakfast? That's a win. Applaud like you've just finished a marathon.

- **Talk to yourself kindly.** When you look in the mirror, resist the urge to launch a verbal assault. Say hello. Thank your body for keeping you upright. Even if it's only just.

- **Ditch toxic comparisons.** You are not the people on Instagram. You are not even the people on your street. You are you – a recovering legend trying to navigate a new world.

Your Friend on the Sofa

The mirror doesn't know everything, indeed it doesn't show you the internal battles – the grit it takes to get through a day, the resilience behind every paced step, every planned nap, every "no" you say for the sake of your health. But **you** know. You live with it every day.

So maybe, just maybe, that person in the mirror isn't a stranger. Perhaps they're a warrior. A bit wrinklier. Possibly fluffier. But stronger in ways no one can see.

Your new self isn't worse. Just different. And deserving of love, patience, and – let's be honest – a few extra naps.

You're doing just fine. Keep going, lovely. You're more *you* than ever.

THE GRIEF YOU DIDN'T EXPECT

When we hear the word "grief," we tend to think of funerals, black suits, and those triangle sandwiches no one enjoys. We think of death, of loss with a capital L. What we rarely talk about is the grief that arrives with chronic illness – the quiet, invisible, endlessly unfolding kind that doesn't come with flowers or sympathy cards.

COVID is a thief in slow motion. It steals energy, confidence, social life, career plans, hobbies, and spontaneity. But more than that, it takes the version of you you used to know—and doesn't return it.

And what follows is grief. Raw, relentless, shapeshifting grief.

The Death of the Before You

There was a version of you before this all began. Maybe you ran half marathons or hoovered without pulling a muscle. Maybe you danced at weddings, pulled all-nighters for work, or wrangled small children without ending up in bed for three days.

And now? You plan your day around how many spoons you have left. You think twice before accepting a coffee invite. You weigh the risk of standing in a queue.

You may not have had a funeral for the before-you, but that doesn't mean they haven't gone. That loss is real. It deserves to be named, honoured, even mourned.

But because you're still here, it confuses people. They think grief is reserved for what's gone entirely. But chronic illness keeps you in a state of ambiguous loss – grieving someone you're still living with.

Grief is Not Linear and Neither is Fatigue

We're sold this tidy narrative of grief: denial, anger, bargaining, depression, acceptance – like a neat little to-do list you can tick off with a biro and a cup of tea. But chronic illness laughs in the face of linear processes.

You may find acceptance one week and be flat on your back in full-blown fury the next. You may feel okay about your limitations in the morning and be in tears by tea time. You might even feel guilty about grieving, because technically, you're "still here."

Grief and Long COVID dance together like drunk cousins at a wedding: awkward, unpredictable, and liable to trip over the buffet table at any moment.

What Are You Grieving Exactly?

Let's spell it out. You might be grieving:

- Your physical abilities

- Your career momentum

- Your independence

- Your social life
- Your hobbies
- Your spontaneity
- Your libido (remember that?)
- Your future as you imagined it
- Your sense of identity

This is not self-pity. This is the truth. And truth, when it's painful, needs space to breathe.

The Loneliness of Unseen Loss

When someone breaks a leg, people rush in with casseroles and well wishes. The silence can be deafening when dealing with Long COVID, which may or may not be visible, understood, or believed.

You learn quickly how to say "I'm fine" when you're not, how to smile through a fog of exhaustion, how to downplay how much you're losing. Because how do you explain that you're grieving a life people think you still have?

The loneliness isn't just physical—it's existential. You are changed, and the world hasn't caught up.

Rage, Sorrow and Suddenly Getting Tearful in the Veg Aisle

Grief doesn't always look like sobbing under a duvet. Sometimes it seems like rage when someone says, "You don't look sick." Sometimes it's despair when you realise you can't do something basic, like carry a bag of shopping, without collapsing later. Sometimes it's weeping in the biscuit aisle because you miss who you used to be.

And it's all valid. Anger, sadness, numbness, bitterness. None of it means you're ungrateful. None of it means you're weak. It means you're human.

WHEN IT ALL GETS A BIT MUCH

Let's not sugarcoat this: living with Long Covid is hard. Relentlessly, invisibly, soul-gnawingly hard. It is a condition that not only hijacks your body but also rewrites your sense of self, erodes your confidence, and pulls at the seams of your mental health until you don't recognise the person staring back at you in the mirror.

And some days are long, grey, and heavy—it all just gets too much.

This section is not here to offer platitudes. You will not find inspirational quotes in cursive fonts. You will find truth—painfully honest, sometimes a bit challenging, but ultimately hopeful truth that has been hard won.

Depression and Long Covid: A Cruel Tag Team

Long Covid is not just a physical illness. It messes with your brain chemistry. It isolates you. It traps you in your own body. It can render you exhausted, foggy, scared, and aching while the world keeps spinning, expecting you to keep up.

It's no surprise, then, that depression becomes a regular and unwelcome houseguest.

Depression doesn't always look like sobbing into your cereal. Sometimes it's numbness. Apathy. The complete absence of joy. Sometimes it's snapping at loved ones and then drowning in guilt. Sometimes it's lying in bed and not brushing your teeth because even that feels like climbing Everest in flip-flops.

And sometimes it's just a quiet voice whispering, "What's the point?"

What Are the Signs?

You may be depressed if you notice:

- You've lost interest in things that once brought joy

- You're sleeping too much or not enough

- You feel hopeless, worthless, or like a burden

- You struggle to make even the smallest decisions

- You have thoughts that scare you

- You feel flat, grey, detached, or overwhelmed

These symptoms can be subtle at first. They can creep in. They can overlap with Long Covid symptoms—fatigue, fog, isolation. But when does your mental health start to feel like an illness in its own right? That's when it's time to listen.

Let's Talk About Help

There is no shame in needing help.

Read that again. Say it out loud.

There is no shame in needing help.

You are not failing. You are not weak. You are not being dramatic. You are a human being trying to cope with a chronic illness that has upended your world. And accepting help is not a sign of defeat. It is a deeply courageous act of self-preservation.

But we know how hard it is.

The Mental Hurdle: Asking for Help

Sitting in a GP surgery and saying, "I'm struggling," can feel more challenging than climbing Everest. Hell, getting to the surgery can feel like you swum and hiked to base camp from Dover. It's even harder than brushing your hair on a bad day. You rehearse the words. You try to convince yourself it's not that bad. You downplay. You say, "I'm just tired," or "I'm fine. Just a bit off."

But inside, you are fraying.

The truth is, you deserve help before you're broken. You deserve help before it all unravels. You don't need to hit rock bottom to justify support.

So what does getting help look like?

The GP Visit: Bravery in Action

You book the appointment. Your heart races. You write down what you want to say, but forget half of it when the doctor asks, "How are things?"

Tell the truth—even just a bit of it.

- "I'm not coping." (Note – there is also something called functional depression, you look put together and like you are coping, but you know deep down you aren't)

- "I've lost interest in everything." (This is the big one – if you feel numb and like you are operating your body like a puppeteer, this is meant by 'lost interest'. Your brain has gone a-waltzing elsewhere.)

- "I feel stuck and low and don't know how to get out of it."

Your GP might ask you to fill in a questionnaire (PHQ-9). It's not a test you can fail. It's a tool to open a conversation.

They might suggest therapy. Medication. Or both.

And that's where the next mental hurdle often looms: antidepressants.

The Antidepressant Debate: Fear vs Fact

Many of us have a knee-jerk reaction to the idea of antidepressants. It might sound like:

- "I should be able to fix this myself."

- "They'll change who I am."

- "I don't want to rely on pills."

- "What if they numb me?"

- "What if people judge me?"

These are valid fears. But they are not always true.

Here's what is true:

If you think of mood as a continuum, or a piece of string, all your emotions happen on that string. Happy is at one end, and sad is at the other. If you won the lottery, you would teeter at one end, just as a bereavement sends you to the other. Each emotion, however, will eventually swing back to the middle of the string. Depression, despite how freely the word is used, is when you drop off the end of the string and you can't get back on without help. Your brain is simply out of spoons on this one. Anti-depressants act as a step ladder to boost you back onto the string.

- Antidepressants can be life-saving, but they will take 2 weeks to make a difference.

- They are not a sign of weakness, but of treatment.

- You are not required to suffer to prove your strength.

- You are allowed to try something that might help. There are many types, and if one doesn't work for you, there is always another to try.

- If you are feeling really unsafe, tell someone and get some help now. Do not wait.

Some people experience side effects. Some try one and don't get on with it. But many find that antidepressants give them a foothold, a bit of clarity, a bit of calm. Enough to start climbing out of the pit.

You don't have to be on them forever. You can always change your mind. But they should never be off the table because of stigma.

Therapy: It's Not Just for Meltdowns

There is no award for suffering in silence. Therapy is not reserved for those at the edge. Therapy is for processing, unpacking, and rebalancing. It is a space where you don't have to pretend.

With Long Covid, therapy can be a vital space to grieve the life you lost. To find language for your anger. To learn how to exist in this new, unreliable body.

What kind of therapy helps?

- **CBT (Cognitive Behavioural Therapy):** Helps challenge negative thinking loops.

- **ACT (Acceptance & Commitment Therapy):** Focuses on accepting what can't be changed and committing to actions that align with your values.

- **Trauma-Informed Therapy:** Crucial if your Long Covid experience involved medical trauma or neglect.

If you don't click with the first therapist you meet, that's okay. Try another. You deserve someone who gets it.

This Is a Huge Adjustment

Let's say it clearly: Chronic illness is a form of loss.

You have lost energy, function, independence, and spontaneity. You may have also lost income, career paths, social connections, and even parts of your identity.

That is grief. That is trauma.

So, of course, it is hard. Of course, you feel low. Of course, you are struggling.

Let's not pathologise what is fundamentally a human reaction to massive, relentless change.

But let's also not pretend you have to weather it alone.

Navigating the Toughest Moments

When it all gets too much, and you find yourself in the pit:

1. **Tell Someone: a** friend, a doctor, a helpline. Speaking the words lifts some of the weight.

2. **Don't Wait for Crisis.** Get help when the early signs appear. Prevention is powerful.

3. **Ground Yourself.** Use simple grounding techniques:

   - Name five things you can see.

   - Touch something cold.

   - Take off your shoes and put your feet flat on the floor.

4. **Make a Safety Plan.** Who will you call? What comforts you? What distracts you safely?

5. **Seek Emergency Help If Needed.** If you have suicidal thoughts or feel unsafe, please get urgent help. You matter. Your story is not finished.

Support That Can Make a Difference

- **Peer Support Groups:** Online or local, these can be lifelines.

- **Mental Health Charities:** Mind, Samaritans, Rethink.

- **Self-Compassion Practices:** Speak to yourself like you would a loved one.

- **Journaling:** This is not for everyone, but writing it out can relieve mental noise.

- **Tiny Joys:** Find a bearable small thing each day, even if it's just stroking a pet or a warm drink.

Your Friend on the Sofa

<u>You Are Still Here</u>

That in itself is an achievement.

Long Covid takes so much. But it cannot take away your right to care. To comfort. To support. To be heard.

Getting help isn't weak. It's the bravest, kindest, most essential thing you can do.

You matter. Your pain matters. Your future still exists.

Let's make sure you're here to see it. Grab a tissue, you're going to be okay.

Fear, Reinfection, and the Eternal Internal Scream

There you are, minding your own business, enjoying a rare public outing. You've dressed like a human, eaten real food, and dared to be in the vicinity of other mammals.

And then it happens.

Someone coughs.

Not just any cough—**a "dry, suspicious, horror-movie-trailer" cough**. Your eyes lock. Your soul screams. You immediately start calculating airflow direction, droplet dispersion, and whether you can plausibly hide under a table without it being too dramatic.

Congratulations. **New fear unlocked: getting Covid again.**

Wait, Can I Actually Get Covid *Again*?

Yes. Yes, you can. We all can. Covid, it turns out, is the clingy ex of viruses—**keeps showing up in your life, completely uninvited**, ignoring all social cues and the fact you've very clearly moved on.

Reinfection is very real. The good news? Most reinfections are *less severe*. The bad news? That's just a statistical average and **you are not a statistic—you are a main character with anxiety and a smartphone**.

If you've had Long Covid, the prospect of being re-infected isn't just a mild concern. It's full-on "pacing-in-the-kitchen-in-your-dressing-gown-like-a-haunted-widow" terror. You've already lost time, energy, and possibly the ability to drink coffee without your heart rate sounding like a rave. Of course you're scared.

Is It Reasonable to Be This Scared?

Yes. But also no. But also yes again. It's complicated.

Let's break it down:

- **Reasonable fear**: You already had a traumatic experience. Your brain is doing its job by saying, "Let's never do that again."

- **Unreasonable-but-deeply-understandable fear**: You now assume every cough, sneeze, or oddly clammy stranger on the train is a direct threat to your life.

- **Borderline apocalyptic fear**: You've started researching how to build your own hermetically sealed bubble out of cling film and optimism.

So yes, it's valid. But the trick is not letting **it drive every decision you make forever**. Fear is like Marmite. A little on the side, fine. But once it's coating everything, it's time for an intervention.

What Do We Actually Know Now?

Let's dive into some facts, with the comforting tone of someone reading a horror novel in a bubble bath.

- **Reinfections are common** now, especially with new variants that are sneaky little buggers. Vaccines wane over time, and variants love a loophole.

- **Most people don't get worse with each reinfection**, but there *is* a small risk that Long Covid could return or be exacerbated.

- **Severity varies**: Some people catch it again and recover in days. Others feel like they've been hit by an IKEA wardrobe of fatigue. It's unpredictable—like British summer.

- **Vaccination helps**. It's not a perfect shield, but it's your best shot (pun very much intended) at reducing severity.

There's no guarantee, but **there never** was, really—not with Covid, and not with life in general.

What If There's Another Pandemic?

Brilliant. That's just what we needed: bonus dread.

Yes, another pandemic is technically possible. We live on a highly connected, slightly soggy planet filled with species that love licking each other's faces and deforesting ecosystems. It's a party out there.

But no, you're probably not going to die. Nottoday. Probably not tomorrow either. Statistically, you're more likely to dieof **googling your symptoms** and spiralling into panic than from the thing you're actually afraid of.

Still, it's not *irrational* to worry. If you've been traumatised by an illness, the world suddenly feels like a place where **death might be hiding behind the next Pret a Manger sneeze guard.**

But—deep breath—**you can't live in that place forever.**

So What Do I Do? Engage with Life or Become a Cryptid?
Here's the crux: **There is no 100% safe option.**

- **Total isolation** is very safe from viruses but very dangerous to your mental health, identity, social connections, and ability to remember how to use a fork in public.

- **Full social reintegration** is risky, exhausting, and full of coughs, but it's also where joy, hugs, art galleries, and crisps in pubs live.

So what's the middle ground?

Sensible, Panicked Precautions:

- **Wear a mask** in high-risk settings. Not a political statement. Just a cloth over your face. Like a ninja, but sadder.

- **Ventilate everything.** Open windows like you're in a Jane Austen novel. Bonus: fresh air, fewer ghosts.

- **Stay up to date on vaccines.** It's a boring adult chore like descaling your kettle, but very worth it.

- **Test if you feel off.** LFTs are still useful. Treat a sore throat like a warning light, not a suggestion.

- **Know your escape routes.** Go to the thing, but give yourself permission to leave early or opt out if your body throws a wobbly.

Most importantly, **choose your risks with intention**. Don't isolate because you're scared. Isolate because you're protecting your energy. Don't go out because you feel forced. Go because you want to. Wanting life doesn't mean you're reckless—it means you're human.

In Summary (Because Long Covid Brains Love a Recap)

- Getting reinfected is possible, but most reinfections are manageable.

- Fear is normal. Living entirely by fear? Not ideal.

- Take reasonable precautions, don't wrap yourself in cling film (unless it's for fun, no judgment).

- Engage with life when and how you can. Even tiny engagements—coffee with a friend, a walk, a laugh—can be acts of glorious rebellion.

You've already survived so much. You don't need to be fearless. You just need to be *brave enough* to keep living.

ASKING FOR HELP

Let's get something straight right off the bat: asking for help is hard. Like, embarrassingly, ego-shatteringly, "rather wrestle a badger than admit I can't carry this box of oat milk" hard. It feels a bit like admitting defeat in the Battle of British Stoicism—a battle in which your Nan, who survived World War II with nothing but a tin of corned beef and quiet judgment, would not approve of your surrender.

But here's the rub: **Long Covid doesn't give a toss about your pride**. It doesn't care that you once lifted a sofa on your own in 2003 or that you "don't like to make a fuss." It just quietly steals your energy, short-circuits your brain, and turns walking up the stairs into an Olympic sport for which you are wildly unqualified.

Pride: Formerly Useful, Now Mostly a Hazard

Pride used to be useful. It got us through job interviews, blind dates, and the horror of admitting we've never actually seen *The Godfather*. But post-Long Covid? Pride becomes about as helpful as a chocolate teapot in a sauna. You end up struggling silently, pretending you're "just a bit tired" when in fact you've had to lie down halfway through brushing your teeth.

Let's put it this way: pride is a luxury. Like boutique gin or shoes that don't hurt. Lovely if you can afford it, but ultimately impractical when you're rationing your energy like a church mouse with a large cheese mortgage.

Asking for Help Without Feeling Like a Failure (Even Though You Secretly Still Will)

The first step to asking for help is accepting that **you need help**. Revolutionary, I know. But there is something oddly terrifying about saying, "Actually, I can't do that today." You worry people will think you're lazy, dramatic, or—worst of all—a Millennial. (Regardless of your actual age.)

But the truth is: **nobody worth knowing will judge you**. And if they do, feel free to cough gently in their direction and walk away.

Some ways to ask for help that don't feel quite so... tragic:

- **The Faux-Casual Text**

    "Hey, any chance you're going to the shops later? Totally fine if not! Just thought I'd check, no pressure, can absolutely crawl there myself."

    (You've still managed to make it sound like you're doing *them* favour.)

- **The Self-Deprecating Plea**

    "Would you mind giving me a hand with dinner? I tried cooking last night and ended up eating crackers in the bath like a sad raccoon."

(Laughter makes it easier. And everyone loves a good sad raccoon visual.)

- **The Honest Approach**

  "I really hate asking, but I'm feeling awful today and I need some help. Would you mind?"

  (Vulnerable, scary, and powerful. Also, if they say no, you're legally allowed to delete them from your Christmas card list.)

But What If They Think I'm a Burden?

Congratulations! You're officially British.

Here's the thing: humans are mostly decent. They want to help. It makes them feel useful, appreciated, and slightly smug in a benevolent way. You know how good it feels to be the person who remembers someone's food allergies at a party? Let them have that moment.

You're not a burden. You're a person experiencing a chronic condition that's about as predictable as a cat on acid. You're managing something huge. And that's enough.

Your Friend on the Sofa

The Sofa of Despair (as I have named it) is the place I do most of my introspection these days. And what I've realised, nestled among crumpled blankets and a half-eaten Digestive, is this:

Pride didn't help me get better. But asking for help? That gave me little glimmers of life back—tiny rebellions against this bastard virus.

So, wave your tiny white flag. Text your mate. Ask your mum to drop off soup. Let someone carry your bags, physically or emotionally.

You'll be amazed at how many people want to help you once you give them permission.

(Just don't expect them to remember your gluten intolerance. Some things never change.)

THE AWKWARD BIT: WHEN OTHERS DON'T GET IT

Nothing like chronic illness to shine a spotlight on who gets it... and who does not. You'll notice friends who vanish, relatives who offer inspirational memes instead of empathy, and colleagues who assume you're on a prolonged holiday.

You may grieve them, too: the faltering friendships, the support that never materialises, and the conversations that feel like performance reviews for your recovery.

It's not just your body that's changed. It's your relationships; navigating that loss can be as painful as anything internally.

Giving Yourself Space

You don't need to "get over it." You're allowed to be sad, to be furious, to lie on the carpet and mutter, "This is bollocks." Because it is.

You're allowed to:

- Cry when you can't do something you used to do effortlessly

- Mourn your energy like an ex you didn't appreciate enough

- Feel envious of joggers and people who can stay out past 9 pm

- Feel joy and grief simultaneously

Permit yourself to feel it all. The sadness, the rage, the fear, the longing – it's not a weakness. It's part of healing, even if your body doesn't cooperate.

Honouring the You That Was

Create your kind of memorial. Write a letter to the old you. Make a photo album. Light a candle. Not because they're gone forever, but because they mattered.

They still matter.

You didn't stop being you. You adapted. You endured. You're still showing up – even if that means shuffling to the kettle and collapsing on the sofa. That counts.

Finding Meaning (Not The Toxic Kind)

Let's be clear: not everything happens for a reason. Some things are just crap.

But meaning can still be made, even in the rubble. Maybe it's finding gentleness you didn't know you had. Maybe it's more profound empathy. Perhaps it's learning to rest without guilt (okay, still working on that one).

There may come a time – not now, maybe not for ages – when you look back and think: That was the hardest thing I ever lived through. But I lived.

Your Friend on the Sofa

<u>You're Still Worthy</u>

Illness doesn't make you less. It doesn't erase your talents, humour, value, or right to take up space – even horizontal- on the good sofa.

Grief doesn't mean you've failed. It means you've loved something deeply enough to feel its loss.

And that? That's brave.

You don't need to do it neatly. Just honestly.

Keep going. You're not alone.

WHO AM I NOW? IDENTITY AND CHRONIC ILLNESS

Y ou don't wake up one morning and think, *"I shall now begin my journey as a person with a chronic illness."* It happens in slow motion, or all at once. And somewhere between the medical appointments, the unanswered questions, and the sudden need to schedule naps like social events, you realise that *my identity has changed.*

But no one tells you how to be this new person. How to navigate the space between who you were and who you're becoming. How can you explain this liminal state to people who still see you as you were, not as you are?

The Awkward Shift in the Mirror

You used to introduce yourself with ease. "I'm a teacher." "I'm a runner." "I'm a parent, a night owl, a reliable friend who brings home-made cakes to meetings." Now, those parts of you might be quiet, distant, or missing altogether.

You might not know what to say when someone asks, *"So what do you do?"* Or worse: *"Are you better yet?"* (Don't worry, we'll get to that bit later.)

Living with Long COVID – or any newly acquired chronic illness – puts your identity into flux. You may feel stuck between versions of yourself—one foot in the past, one foot on a banana peel.

When People Start Seeing You Differently

There's a subtle shift in how people respond to you once you're no longer entirely well. They may speak to you more slowly or more loudly. They may ask fewer questions about your life or offer unsolicited advice instead of genuine curiosity.

Or they may quietly disappear, unsure how to relate to you now. (Spoiler: that says more about them than it does about you.)

And sometimes, you start to internalise these changed perceptions. *Maybe I'm not capable anymore. Perhaps I am just a patient now.* This, friends, is where internalised ableism often begins to creep in.

Ableism and the Invisibility Cloak

Ableism is the assumption that being able-bodied is the default, and that those who aren't are somehow lesser. It's everywhere: in architecture, employment policies, inspirational memes about "overcoming disability." And if your disability or chronic illness is invisible, as Long COVID often is, the gaslighting can be even worse.

You may feel pressure to "look well" to avoid judgment, only to be dismissed or doubted because you *look* well. It's a lose-lose dance choreographed by other people's assumptions.

But the most challenging part? Ableism isn't just out there – it's often in us, too.

We might tell ourselves:

- "I'm not disabled, I'm just struggling."

- "I don't want to be one of those people."

- "If I just try harder, maybe I'll get back to normal."

You can be exactly as you are, without explaining, performing, or proving anything to anyone.

Disability Identity: Embrace, Reject, or Reframe?

For some, claiming the identity of "disabled" is powerful. It opens doors to legal protections, community, and a language for experiences that previously felt isolating. It's not about defeat – it's about recognition.

For others, the word feels uncomfortable, like it doesn't fit, or they fear what embracing it might mean. Long COVID, especially, is unpredictable. No one knows if it's forever, fixable, or something in between. Are we just passing through?

There is no single right way to navigate this. It's okay to see disability as a part of who you are. It's also okay to see it as a temporary condition or a frustrating mystery that refuses to be pinned down. Identity is personal. It's not a team sport.

But here's what's vital: **don't tear each other down over labels**. Whether someone chooses to use the word "disabled," "chronically ill," "energy limited," "fatigued AF," or "person with Long COVID," we are all describing the same storm – we're just choosing different umbrellas.

The Myth of Getting Back to Normal

Everyone wants to know when you're getting back to normal. It's a question disguised as encouragement but often laced with discomfort: *Please recover quickly so we can all stop being reminded that bodies are fragile.*

But what if there's no "back" to go to? What if you're building something entirely new – even if it's made out of pacing charts, disability benefits forms, and more pillboxes than a pharmacy?

Reclaiming identity doesn't mean going backwards. It means finding who you are in this new shape and reality.

Fitting Into the World Again (Or Not)

You may feel like you've been shoved to the margins of work, social life, and visibility. You might not be able to keep up, or you might not even be able to show up.

And yet, you are still here. You still belong. Your value is not in what you produce or how reliably you show up to brunch.

Creating identity in chronic illness is not about pretending to be the old you. It's about expanding what it means to be *you*, period.

You may now be:

- A person who rests unapologetically

- Someone who advocates for accessibility

- A friend who shows up emotionally, even when your body can't

- A master of boundaries

- A survivor in every sense

And that's not less than. It's simply *different*.

Community Over Division

As the Long COVID and chronic illness communities grow, there's a risk of fragmentation: camps forming around language, prognosis, and identity. Those who identify as disabled. Those who don't. Those who seek cures. Those who focus on acceptance. But we can't afford to fracture.

Every lived experience is valid. We need **all** of us:

- The hopeful

- The uncertain

- The angry

- The adapting

- The deeply, gloriously exhausted

We are stronger together, not despite our different paths, but because of them.

If we can hold space for each other—without judgment or agenda—we might find a kind of identity that doesn't shrink us but *includes* us.

Your Friend on the Sofa
<u>You're Still You</u>

Chronic illness may change how you move through the world. It may change what you can do, how others see you, and how you see yourself. But it does not erase your core.

You are still funny, kind, clever, grumpy, creative, tender, opinionated, and resilient. You are still someone worth knowing, listening to, and loving.

And you're still becoming. You don't need to have it all figured out. Just take your time. Breathe. Try the labels on or throw them out. There's no quiz at the end.

You are not broken. You are unfolding.

THE ROLE OF THE PATIENT

Let's get one thing straight: there is no *correct* way to be a patient or disabled.

There is, however, a suspiciously persistent myth floating about – a sort of social script – that tells us how we *should* behave. Be compliant. Be grateful. Be gentle. Be humble. Be tragically brave, but never too loud about it. And whatever you do, don't get angry because an angry patient is a *non-compliant* patient.

Let's burn that script, shall we?

The Problem with the Patient Performance

Somewhere along the line, we decided that sick people should become meek, mild, pliable versions of themselves. Bonus points if they're inspirational while doing it.

Smile politely through the tests. Accept the meds with a grateful nod. Never question a doctor. Never roll your eyes at your fourth waiting room delay. Never dare to express the tiniest flicker of fury at the injustice of it all. Because if you do? You're difficult. You're problematic. You're *non-compliant*.

Here's a radical idea: **you are allowed to be furious.** You might be a fully three-dimensional human who is ill *and* still has a spine.

The Myth of the Deserving Sick

A noxious little societal myth suggests that only the "deserving" should get care, sympathy, or even the right to exist loudly. The deserving sick are quiet. Noble. Sad-eyed, pale-skinned saints who've renounced pleasure, lipstick, and carbs. They do not go to parties. They certainly do not wear statement shoes.

Spoiler: this myth is bollocks.

Chronic illness does not handpick the pious. It does not reward good behaviour. It does not care if you recycle, meditate, or were mean to your cousin at Christmas. You can be good, bad, flawed, chaotic, glamorous, grumpy, kind, funny, furious, or above.

Illness is not a moral judgement.

So why do we act like being sick requires a personality transplant or scramble back into our past to find out what we did that was so heinous to deserve this?

You Don't Have to Rebrand

Here's the good news: you don't have to change who you are to be a patient. You don't have to bleach your personality to fit into a hospital gown.

- If you were funny, bold, a bit inappropriate, and deeply sarcastic before your diagnosis, good news, you still get to be all of those things.

- Keep going if you were loud, passionate, and had an outfit for every mood.

- If you were prickly and needed therapy before... well, that's still highly recommended, but not because of your illness.

You get to be fully, unapologetically *you*. Hanging onto that identity might be the thing that keeps you sane.

The Word We Hate: Non-Compliant

Ah, yes, "non-compliant" – the word that says more about the healthcare system than it does about the patient. In theory, it refers to someone who doesn't follow medical advice. In practice, it often gets slapped onto anyone who:

- Asks too many questions

- Has a complicated case

- Refuses to go away when the medical profession doesn't have an answer at the moment

- Doesn't respond to treatment in a textbook way or fits onto an established pathway

- Advocates for themselves

- Gets angry

- Dresses fabulously

You are not a bad patient because you expect dignity and clarity, or refuse to whisper your truth through gritted teeth.

Compliance isn't the goal. *Collaboration* is.

Here's the secret: Your care should always be a partnership with the medical professionals you work with. You are the expert in your condition and anyone telling you what to do or dictating things to you is not following the training. Clinicians, like anyone, can be brilliant but can also be twats.

You Can Be Angry – And Still Be Doing Everything Right
You can be blisteringly, blisteringly furious at being ill and still:

- Take your meds

- Attend appointments

- Try every sodding protocol thrown your way

- Treat clinicians with courtesy

- Be actively working toward managing your health

Anger doesn't negate effort. It doesn't make you ungrateful. It makes you *human*. It's rational to be enraged at the chaos Long COVID (or any chronic condition) has caused.

Anger might be the most appropriate response. Who wouldn't be mad when their body suddenly becomes a full-time job with no salary, sick leave, or HR support?

Responsibility and Rights – They Still Apply
Chronic illness might shift your day-to-day, but it doesn't revoke your autonomy. You still have:

- The right to be treated respectfully

- The right to ask for second opinions

- The right to refuse treatment

- The right to speak up if you're not being heard
- The right to be your whole self, with all the moods and opinions that come with it
- But you also have the responsibility to also not be a twat.

Being ill doesn't remove your voice. It means you may need to use it more, and sometimes more loudly.

And If You Were a Dick Before...

Look, let's be real. If you were rude, entitled, and insufferable before illness, you don't get a free pass now. Chronic illness isn't a personality cleanser.

But for the rest of us – the flawed, kind, feisty, sarcastic, weird, wonderful humans doing their best – you don't have to perform sainthood to be taken seriously.

You are not a patient archetype. You are a person with a complex, valid, and vivid life.

Your Friend on the Sofa

<u>Take Up Space</u>

So, what is the role of the patient?

It's not to be small, silent, or sweet. It's not to be grateful for crumbs. It's not to smile through gritted teeth and nod at every suggestion.

The role of the patient is to survive—on your terms, to collaborate, not obey, to rest, rage, recover, and relapse—all while maintaining your glorious selfhood.

So go on. Wear the red lipstick. Ask the hard questions. Swear under your breath. Show up fully.

You are more than allowed. You are *necessary*.

GOD FORBID I LAUGH

So you've done it.

You've emerged from your bed like a majestic, wobbly phoenix. You've brushed your teeth, put on Real Clothes (by which I mean: not pyjamas with pasta on them), and now—brace yourself—**you're having a laugh.**

You're smiling. You might even be outside. There's music. There's sunlight. Someone dares to comment:

"Wow, you're looking well! Does this mean you're better?"

And just like that, your joy is mugged in a public square.

Chronic Illness and the Great Joy Guilt Trip

Having a chronic illness is a bit like being given a lifetime membership to a club you never joined, where every time you smile someone pops up to remind you:

"You're not supposed to be enjoying yourself, are you?"

As if suffering must always be visible. As if fun invalidates your pain. As if laughing means you've somehow faked the last 18months of lying down and crying into a stale Hobnob.

Let's be clear: **you're allowed to feel joy even when you're unwell**.

You're not faking being sick. You're faking being okay. And frankly, you deserve an award for it.

"But You Were Just at the Pub!"

Yes, and you were just at your niece's soft play birthday party dressed as a frog, Susan, but I'm not accusing you of being professionally amphibious.

Joy is not a metric for health. It is not proof you're "over it." You might laugh uproariously one minute and crash so hard the next you end up horizontal for 48 hours, contemplating mortality and the fluff on your ceiling. This is the chronic illness dance. Two steps forward, one back, a nap in a bin.

And guess what? **That laugh was still worth it**.

The Visibility Problem

People like illness to come with visible clues: casts, bandages, maybe a faint wan face and a tragic violin soundtrack. But chronic illness is sneaky. It's internal. It's invisible.

So when people see you laughing or dancing or enjoying an aggressively overpriced oat milk latte, they assume you're cured.

They don't see you:
- Crawling into bed after

- Canceling everything the next day

- Crying quietly because your body betrayed you again

But you see it. And that's enough.

Joy Is Medicine (And It's Free, Mostly)

Here's the radical idea: **fun is good for you.**

Laughter lowers stress. Joy calms the nervous system. A moment of delight can be the difference between "barely coping" and "okay, maybe I can face the world again."

Think of joy as physical therapy for your spirit. And no, you don't need to earn it. You don't need to be well enough, productive enough, or "sick enough" to deserve a good time.

If you want to sing off-key to 2006 bangers in your living room while sitting down—**you absolutely should.**

If you manage to go out and laugh till your face hurts and then spend the next two days in bed—**that doesn't mean you messed up.** That means you lived. And it was beautiful.

Dealing with "Well-Meaning" Comments

Some scripts, for your next encounter with someone whose mouth moves faster than their empathy:

- **"You look better!"**

  "Oh thank you! I'm still sick, but this is a rare 'upright' day. Cherish it."

- **"So... are you back to normal now?"**

  "Sort of! If normal includes napping like a cat and needing six hours to digest a sandwich.

- **"You can't be that ill if you're out, can you?"**

  "You can't be that rude if you're speaking, can you?" (Use sparingly. Or frequently. Dealer's choice.)

Your Friend on the Sofa

You are a whole person. Not just a diagnosis. And whole people laugh. They cry, they love, they binge terrible TV, they post memes, they find reasons to keep going.

Chronic illness doesn't cancel your right to joy—**it makes it more necessary**.

So laugh. Giggle like a misbehaving child. Flirt with the barista. Go to the gig. Say yes to the picnic. Make the joke.

Your body might be broken, but your joy? Your joy is defiant.

And there's something a little bit punk rock about laughing in the face of something that tried to take everything from you.

(Just remember to bring a blanket, a snack, and possibly a friend to carry you home after.)

Part Four - Summary for the Foggy.

- **Who Is That in the Mirror?**: Long Covid can turn your reflection into a stranger. Bloating, dark circles, and the "permanently exhausted pigeon" look are now part of the aesthetic.

- **Body Betrayal 101**: Your limbs are moody, your joints are traitors, and your stamina ghosted you. It's like your body's on strike and forgot to tell you.

- **Weighty Issues**: Whether you've gained or lost weight, your body feels unfamiliar. And no, unsolicited advice is *not* helpful and kale is still awful.

- **Confidence = Stolen**: Illness doesn't just steal energy; it nicks your swagger too. You're still you—just under layers of symptoms, pyjamas, and existential dread.

- **Making Peace with Your Meat Suit**: Talk to your body like it's a grumpy roommate. Celebrate tiny wins. Wear the comfy clothes. Ditch comparisons. Love the you that exists *now*.

- **Grieving the 'Before You'**: No one threw a funeral, but you've lost a version of yourself—and that loss is real. Grief isn't linear. It's messy, exhausting, and totally valid.

- **Invisible Grief Is Still Grief**: People may not *see* what you've lost. But you do. That silent mourning? It matters. You're grieving a life others assume you still live.

- **Depression and Long Covid: Tag-Team Hell**: Brain fog, numbness, sadness, snapping at your loved ones. If joy feels out of reach, you're not broken—you're struggling, and that's okay.

- **Ask for Help (Before It All Unravels)**: Whether it's therapy, medication, or just telling someone you're not okay—asking for support is strength, not failure.

- **Antidepressants Aren't the Enemy**: They're not mind control. They're a ladder out of the pit. If your brain's out of spoons, medication might just be the boost you need.

- **Therapy = Mental Maintenance**: You don't need to be on the brink to benefit. You're not weak for needing support—you're wise for seeking it.

- **Joy Guilt Is a Scam**: Just because you laughed doesn't mean you're cured. Joy is not a symptom of wellness—it's a victory. And yes, it's still worth the crash.

- **Joy Is Resistance**: Laughter, memes, 2006 bangers—whatever brings you joy is medicine. You're allowed to live, to laugh, and to feel human again (even if it costs you a two-day recovery).

- **Final Word**: You are not lazy. You are not broken. You are surviving something massive. And if you smiled today—even once—that's radical defiance. Keep going.

"My lungs wheeze like an asthmatic accordion, and my brain fog is thicker than a Real Housewife's foundation"

Part Five - WTF do I say?

Ah yes. The dreaded line. The verbal equivalent of a wet flannel to the face: "But you look fine." Usually said with wide-eyed optimism, as if they've just solved your health mystery with a compliment. Spoiler: they haven't. Let's get this out of the way — looking and being fine are very different. And if looking ill were a prerequisite for being treated with compassion, most of us would need to drag around an oxygen tank, two crutches, and wear a sign saying "Please ask me about my internal suffering."

So, what do you say when someone hits you with this unintentional microaggression?

Let's explore with some more sassy answers. I go for full drag queen burn and then tone them down a bit, but my goodness, there is something satisfying about writing them down.

But you don't *look* sick!"

- "And you don't look medically qualified, but here you are giving diagnoses with your dusty little opinion."

- "What do you want, a tragic filter and a fog machine?"

- "I don't *look* sick? It's called concealer and trauma bonding with my mirror."

"Are you sure it's not just stress?"
"Yes. And I'm also sure it's not caused by talking to people like you."
"No, stress is what I feel when someone with the IQ of a biscuit tries to talk science."
"Yes, I was so stressed I decided to disable myself for the aesthetic."

"Have you tried yoga/green juice/waking up earlier?"

- "Yes, and I still want to slap you with a rolled-up yoga mat."

- "If yoga could cure this, I'd do downward dog while levitating round the room."

- "Oh yes, I tried juicing — my will to live. Didn't help."

"Maybe you're just tired like the rest of us."

- "Oh, your version of tired is my pre-warmup for catastrophic collapse."

- "You're tired? I run on three brain cells and a prayer — don't test me."

- "Darling, if you felt what I feel, you'd be horizontal and crying into oat milk."

"I had Covid too, and I was fine!"
- "Congrats. You want a sash or just attention?"
- "Wow, you survived a different illness. That's like bragging you didn't drown in someone else's pool."
- "And I ate a peanut and didn't die. Should I call every allergic person a liar?"

"But you were fine yesterday!"
- "And you had dignity yesterday. See how quickly things change?"
- "Yesterday was the preview. Today's the horror sequel."
- "Yes, I borrowed one functioning day. The interest rate was hell."

"It's probably just anxiety."
- "Yes, I'm so anxious my immune system threw a rave in my bloodstream."
- "Oh sure, I'll just manifest a normal nervous system like you manifested a personality."
- "You're right. I'm just so dramatic, I faint for character development."

"Maybe if you were healthier, you wouldn't have Long Covid."
- "Oh, sweetie, the virus didn't ask for my smoothie preferences before wrecking my organs."

- "I was healthy, then I got Covid. You were ignorant, and somehow *still* are."

- "It's not a lifestyle issue. It's a *you having no empathy* issue."

"You just don't want to get better."
- "Yes, I'm deeply committed to a life of naps and explaining my existence to clowns like you."

- "Of course, I live for the glamour of symptom spreadsheets and being horizontal by noon."

- "I don't want to get better? Honey, I'd sell your soul for a normal immune response."

Final Word for All the Above:
- "I'm not saying you're medically illiterate, but if I threw your opinion in the bin, even the germs would say 'pass.'"

- "Long Covid is real. Your grasp on reality? Not so much."

- "Go commune with a shrub. Preferably far away from me."

Your Friend on the Sofa

A Tiny Bit of Empathy (Even If It's Hard)

Most people aren't trying to be hurtful. They genuinely don't understand what it means to live with an invisible illness. They've been conditioned to equate wellness with aesthetics. (Thanks, Instagram.) Sometimes, the best we can do is educate. Or at least inform with a sharp, but funny, retort. Either way, you've got options. And just because you "look fine" doesn't mean you must accept their misunderstanding as a compliment. You are not a fraud. You are not overreacting. You are surviving. And looking good while doing it. If you want to spend some time moisturising or applying makeup, that is your business, so go for it.

HOW TO EXPLAIN LONG COVID WITHOUT SCREAMING INTO A PLANT

So, Someone asks:

"What exactly *is* Long Covid?"

Depending on who's asking, your instinct may vary wildly:

- You want to give them a TED Talk with graphs.

- You want to cry.

- You want to laugh darkly and say, "It's like getting trampled by a slow-motion elephant for 600 days."

- You want to hide under a duvet and pretend you didn't hear the question.

Let's break it down. There are many kinds of listeners, and many kinds of answers. You get to choose your adventure.

Listener Type 1: The Kind But Confused
They say: "Wow, you're still not better?" or "I thought Covid was just like the flu?"
How to reply:
"I had a mild case of Covid. But for some people, the virus triggers something long-term in the body. It messes with systems — immune, nervous, cardiovascular. Some people recover. Some don't. I'm one of the 'don't'... at least for now."
Add if you like:
"It's kind of like my body is running on dial-up internet, in 2025. Some days I can do a thing. Then I can't. My energy resets weirdly. It's not just 'tired' — it's broken operating system vibes."

Listener Type 2: The Minimiser
They say: "We're *all* tired." "Have you tried pushing through?" "My neighbour cured it with goat yoga and celery."
You think: I want to yeet myself into the sun.
Try this:
"I get that. This isn't just tired. It's a medical condition with inflammation, immune disruption, and sometimes damage to the heart or brain. If I do too much, I crash. Like, can't-speak, can't-move crash. It's not just about 'needing a rest.' It's a whole systemic issue."
Optional bonus line, delivered calmly but firmly:
"And honestly, the 'have you tried' suggestions can feel invalidating. I know you mean well. But I'm managing this with my medical team. And my snacks."

Listener Type 3: The Genuinely Worried
They say: "Oh my god — are you dying?" "You look... okay?" *(said like a question)* "Is it contagious?"

How to comfort them without becoming their therapist:
"I'm not dying. But I am living with something chronic and complicated. Some people do recover. Some of us learn to manage it, like any long-term condition. It's not contagious anymore — it's just my body being confused about how to function."

Bonus reassurance:
"You don't need to treat me like I'm fragile, but maybe don't expect me to dance through brunch. Just being here is me winning."

Listener Type 4: The Slightly Hostile/Disbelieving
They say: "It's all in your head, though, right?" "My cousin had that, and she's fine now." "Don't you think you're focusing on it too much?"

You *could* scream. Or...
"There's a growing pile of research showing Long Covid affects multiple systems in the body. It's not just mood or mindset. And if it *were* in my head, mental health conditions still deserve care and support. But this is very much in my body."

Add if necessary (and you've had enough):
"If you don't understand, that's okay. But please don't dismiss it just because it's invisible. If you saw my blood results, scans, or the number of specialists I've met, you'd know I'm not exaggerating."

Listener Type 5: The Overreacting/ Germaphobe

They say: "What's wrong with you?" (followed by dramatic side-stepping)"Oh no, is it still Covid??" "Should I be worried? I've got kids."(backs away like you just coughed up plague mist)

You say (as dryly as possible):

"Nope. Not infectious. Not shedding the virus and just managing a post-viral condition. Think about long-term effects, not active germs. You're safer standing next to me than at your kid's school pick-up queue."

Optional extra for maximum sass:

"If I were contagious, I'd be home, not standing here explaining basic immunology to someone treating me like a walking Petri dish." Or :"If this were contagious two years after the fact, the government would've done something about it."

Pro tip: Smile sweetly while saying this. Passive-aggressive sparkle is your best friend here.

How to Explain It Without Burning Out

You don't have to give everyone the whole story. You can create tiers, like a cake.

- **Tier 1 (polite public):** "I've got Long Covid — it affects my energy and nervous system. It's a bit unpredictable, but I'm managing."

- **Tier 2 (curious but not close):** "Some days I can do things. Some days I crash. It's like my body has a weird glitchy operating system. I have to pace everything."

- **Tier 3 (trusted people):** Go deeper. Talk about PEM, brain fog, scary heart palpitations, the whole disco of symptoms.

Let them into your reality, if you want to.

And if someone says, "But you look fine!" you can smile sweetly and say:

"Thank you. That's because you're not seeing me in bed two hours later, wondering if I overdid it by making toast."

Final Note: You Don't Owe Everyone an Explanation

It's not your job to educate the entire planet. But if you choose to — that's brave and generous. If you don't have the energy? That's also completely valid.

Your Friend on the Sofa

"I'd love to explain more, but I'm low on spoons today. Happy to send you something to read later."(Then send them *any part of this book*.)

And remember: You are not weak for being ill. You are not rude for setting boundaries. You are not responsible for fixing anyone's ignorance.

You're just trying to live inside a body that doesn't always cooperate. And that's more than enough.

Conversations That Matter: Talking to Your People

Living with Long Covid is a bit like being handed a script to a play no one else has read. You're trying to act out your part—foggy, flaring, fluctuating—while everyone else carries on in the background, assuming it's business as usual. The lights are too bright, your costume doesn't fit, and the stage is on fire.

Social life doesn't stop for chronic illness, but it changes. Drastically.

This part is about navigating relationships with friends, family, colleagues, partners, and even kids when your capacity has been drastically redefined, but expectations haven't.

Talking to Parents

This one can be the most emotional. Parents want to fix things. They want you well. They may not understand what "no cure yet" means when they only want to swoop in with soup and solve it.

Try saying, "Mum/Dad, I know how much you care. But this isn't going away quickly. I need you to believe me when I say I'm doing everything I can, even if you can't see it. I need your support more than your solutions right now."

Set boundaries gently: "It means a lot that you want to help. I need [help with groceries/quiet time/a chat without advice]."

Talking to Siblings

Siblings can be tricky—they remember the 'you' from before. They might joke, downplay, or avoid the subject altogether.

Try this approach: "I know this all seems weird and different. It is. I still want to be part of your life but might need to do things differently. Can we find ways to stay close that don't need loads of energy from me?"

Make it real for them: "Imagine waking up with the flu and jet lag every day, and still being expected to act normal. That's what this feels like."

Talking to Friends

Some friends get it. Others don't. And it hurts when they don't—especially the ones who once shared your laughter, chaos, and 2 am texts.

Open the door with honesty: "I know I've changed. I miss things too. I'd love to keep our connection, even if that looks different now. Can we start with short catch-ups or voice notes?"

For those who mean well but miss the mark: "I appreciate you checking in. When you say [insert unhelpful comment], I feel misunderstood. I need you just to be there; no fixes are needed."

Talking to a Partner

Chronic illness in a relationship exposes every crack and strengthens every strong beam. It's intimacy redefined: trust, caregiving, and adjusting together.

Try saying: "This is hard for me. I hate what it's doing to us, too. But I'm still here. I still love you. I can't always show it the same way."

Check-ins matter: "Can we talk about how we're both coping with this? I know it affects you too. I want to keep being a team, even if it's slower-paced."

Reassure without pretending: "This isn't the life we planned. But I want to keep building one with you—even if it's got more rest days and fewer restaurant nights."

Talking to Children

Honesty matters. So does simplicity. Kids sense more than we realise.

For younger children: "You know how phones run out of charge and need plugging in? My body is like that. I need more time to rest and recharge, but it's not because I don't want to play."

For older children or teens: "I know it's hard to see me like this. It's hard to be like this. I'm still your parent and love you just as much. I'm learning how to do things differently now."

Let them in gently: "You can always ask questions. You can always tell me how you feel. We're all figuring this out together."

Talking to Your Boss and Colleagues

Work can be one of the most daunting places to explain Long Covid. It requires walking the fine line between honesty, professionalism, vulnerability, and boundaries.

Start with the facts: "I want to be transparent about something important. I have Long Covid, a chronic condition that affects my energy levels, cognitive function, and ability to recover from activity. While I may appear fine, I work with significantly reduced capacity."

Set realistic expectations: "I want to continue contributing to the team, but may need some flexibility. That could look like remote work, flexible hours, or a reduced workload depending on the day."

Give them something to work with: "Some days I'm functional. Other days I'm not. It's not about attitude or effort but about how my body and brain function. I'm happy to keep communicating honestly to find a way."

For colleagues who just don't get it: "I know I don't look sick, and I might even seem normal for a while, but Long Covid is a relapsing-remitting condition. It means my symptoms fluctuate, and if I push too hard, I crash. It's not laziness—it's biology."

Scripts for navigating awkward moments:
- "I'm pacing myself today, so I'll need to take a break after this meeting."

- "I've had a tough flare this week so that I might be a little slower replying. Thanks for your patience."

- "I can't make the after-work drinks, but I'd love to catch up one-on-one sometime."

Use support systems: If your workplace has HR or an occupational health team, involve them. You don't have to navigate this alone. Bring documentation, GP letters, or symptom diaries. They help ground your experience in evidence and reduce the emotional load of constantly explaining yourself.

> **Your Friend on the Sofa**
> Most importantly, remember this: Needing accommodations doesn't make you a liability. It makes you a human being in need of support. It doesn't mean you're not capable. It means you're managing more than most while still showing up. That's courage. That's resilience. And that's worth respecting.

Part Five - Summary for the Foggy.

- **"But You Look Fine" = Verbal Juice Cleanse**: Unwanted, vaguely offensive, and based on vibes not science. Illness ≠aesthetics.

- **Invisible ≠ Imaginary**: Just because you're upright, moisturised, and possibly wearing mascara doesn't mean your nervous system isn't on fire.

- **Comebacks on Standby**: From drag-level burns ("you don't look medically qualified") to sassy sighs ("it's called concealer and despair"), you've got options.

- **Explaining Long Covid Without Crying in a Plant Pot**: Choose-your-own-response depending on whether they're kind, clueless, minimising, panicked, or just plain rude. Spoiler: you owe no TED Talk.

- **Talking to Loved Ones Without Exploding**: Parents want to fix. Siblings may joke. Friends disappear or surprise you. Partners wobble. Kids just want the truth in gentle doses.

- **Work Scripts That Keep You Sane**: "I have a chronic condition, not an attitude problem." "I'm pacing, not slacking." "Yes, I'm sick *and* professional. Wild, right?"

- **Setting Boundaries ≠ Being Rude**: You can say "I'm low on spoons, not on intelligence. Happy to send you something to read instead of performing."

- **To the Germaphobes and Drama Queens**: No, you're not contagious. Yes, they can stop sidestepping you like you're a walking plague cloud. Please sit down.

- **Final Thought**: You're not dramatic. You're chronically ill. You're not overreacting. You're adapting. You're not rude for setting boundaries—you're brilliant for surviving in a world that still expects you to sprint while you're crawling.

> "Long COVID?
> Honey, I've had relationships shorter than this virus.
> At least the virus calls back — your date didn't."

Part Six - HTF Do I Keep Going?

P*acing*
Not a Fun Run, Sadly

Let's get something straight: pacing is not trendy Pilates. It's not a light jog around the park. And it's not code for watching daytime telly while occasionally checking your FitBit. In the context of Long Covid, pacing is a carefully orchestrated act of energy micromanagement that is so advanced that it should come with a spreadsheet and a life coach.

What Is Pacing?

Pacing is the art of doing just enough and not a smidge more. It means planning your activity so you don't end up slumped in a chair with the vitality of a dying houseplant. It's about staying within your energy envelope — yes, that's a real term. Think of it like a mobile data plan: go over your limit, and the consequences are both painful and expensive (except instead of extra charges, you get three days in bed and the crushing guilt of having used a Hoover).

The Energy Envelope

Your energy envelope is the energy you can use daily without triggering Post-Exertional Malaise (PEM). Picture a battery that doesn't fully recharge overnight. Now imagine that battery powers your entire existence, including your ability to make toast or send a text. That's what we're working with. The aim? Stay inside the envelope. Don't try to prove a point to your neighbours by mowing the lawn.

According to Occupational Therapy (OT) guidance:
- Break tasks into chunks. (Brushing your teeth can be a two-part event.)
- Rest before you feel tired. Revolutionary, we know.
- Use tools like timers and alarms to manage activity.
- Prioritise, plan, pace. The holy trinity of chronic illness management. It's not glamorous, but it works.

Pacing isn't giving up. It's giving yourself a fighting chance.

Heart Rate Monitoring – Not Just for Gym Bros

One popular pacing method involves keeping your heart rate below a certain threshold, calculated using the Karvonen formula or subtracting 15 beats per minute from your max aerobic threshold (often around 60% of your age-adjusted max heart rate). It doesn't sound very easy. That's because it isn't. But there are apps and gadgets to help: smartwatches, chest straps, or just checking your pulse the old-fashioned way while pretending you're an 18th-century poet.

Visible has picked up much 'pace' in the community. You can download the app for free or pay for additional monitoring equipment and access if you feel flush. It monitors heart rate, heart rate value continually and transfers these into 'pace scores' which show you how your doing and what activities cost you the most energy. It also provides symptoms trackers and the chance to be in studies to add to the knowledge of professionals for the future.

Breathwork

But Without the Spiritual Overtones (Unless That's Your Thing)

Let's face it: telling someone with Long Covid to "just breathe" is about as helpful as telling a drowning person to "try swimming better." However, there is good evidence that targeted breathing exercises can help with breathlessness, anxiety, and even fatigue. And you don't need to sit on a Himalayan mountaintop or wear Lululemon.

Diaphragmatic Breathing: The Real MVP

Diaphragmatic (or belly) breathing helps reset your nervous system, get oxygen into your bloodstream more efficiently, and calm the fight-or-flight chaos. Here's how you do it:

- Lie down or sit comfortably.

- Place one hand on your chest, the other on your belly.

- Inhale slowly through your nose so your belly rises.

- Exhale through pursed lips, like you're blowing out a tiny birthday candle.

- Repeat.

- <u>Feel smug</u>

Do this for 5-10 minutes, 2-3 times daily. Studies suggest it helps manage dyspnea (a fancy word for breathlessness).

Buteyko Breathing: Not a Pasta Dish
Developed by a Ukrainian doctor, the Buteyko method focuses on reducing over-breathing. Some research suggests it helps with asthma, and it's also being explored for Long COVID.
- Short nasal inhalation

- Gentle nasal exhalation

- Pause before the next breath.

It's technical, but plenty of free YouTube guides are available. Just avoid the ones promising spiritual awakenings and a third eye.

Other Tips:
- Try humming (stimulates the vagus nerve)

- Blow bubbles or use a pinwheel (seriously, it works)

- Use breathing apps with calming visuals.

Bonus: it's free, you can do it in bed, and you won't need a prescription. Just don't let the dog judge you.

Exercise

I Just Walked to the Kettle and Needed a Nap

Ah, yes, the E-word. Once a source of smugness or guilt, now a terrifying proposition that risks a multi-day crash. Let's Revisit PEM (Yes, Again)PEM means your body responds to exertion as if it's been betrayed. When you try to exercise, your system panics like someone who's been asked to host Question Time with no prep. For Long Covid folks, the old "push through" advice is about as useful as a chocolate teapot.

Graded Exercise Therapy (GET): No Thanks

Once the go-to for ME/CFS, GET fell out of favour after research showed it made many patients worse. The updated NICE guidelines (2021) now warn against using it for post-viral fatigue. So no, your cousin's advice to "just do Couch to 5K" is unhelpful and dangerous.

What Actually Helps?

- Stretching: Gentle, controlled, non-aerobic movements

- Rehab with a specialist: Someone who gets post-viral illness

- Pacing: (Yes, again.)

- Strength-building (in tiny increments): Using resistance bands while seated

- Start low, go slow. If in doubt, don't. It's better to miss one session than spend the weekend in bed.

Siesta or Crash?

There comes a time in every Long COVID survivor's journey when the body quietly whispers, "Lie down or perish." Of course, Britain doesn't take kindly to that sort of nonsense. Lying down during the day? What are we, Spanish? Relaxed? Happy?

We've built a whole empire on clenching our teeth and soldiering on, by Jove! Resting in the middle of the day smacks of decadence. Lazy, even. That's something for pensioners, cats, and toddlers. Certainly not for proud, tax-paying Brits with stiff upper lips and bad backs.

But here's the kicker: your mitochondria didn't get the memo about your Protestant work ethic. They are knackered. And unless you start treating your body like the fragile, unpredictable, occasionally malfunctioning jalopy that it now is, you will crash. Hard. Possibly on your neighbour's hydrangeas. Perhaps while holding a scalding cup of tea. Either way, it won't be elegant

The Spanish Secret: The Guilt Free Nap

Let's take a moment to tip our sunhat to our Mediterranean cousins. In Spain, napping is an art form. A siesta is not a sign of weakness. It's a badge of sanity. A cultural institution. Something people plan for, like lunch, or watching their football team disappoint them again. The Spaniards aren't ashamed of napping; they're organised about it. It's not crashing – it's orchestrated energy management. And crucially, no one is made to feel like a Victorian consumptive just because they need forty winks before dinner.

Meanwhile, in Britain, if you fall asleep on the sofa before 8 pm, someone will throw a cushion at your face and shout "wakey wakey, we're not having a lie-in!" – as though lying down might somehow encourage your organs to stage a walkout.

Pacing Rest vs Crash Napping

Here's the meat: when dealing with Long COVID, there are naps and crash naps.

Crash Nap (noun): An unplanned collapse, often following a misguided burst of energy or, God forbid, a short walk to the post box. Usually accompanied by groaning, drooling, and the faint smell of regret.

Planned Nap (noun): A scheduled, gentle rest undertaken before predicted tiredness, often with a blanket, soothing sounds, and the smugness of someone who knows their limits.

The key difference? Control and dignity. A crash nap is when your body goes rogue, throws up the "Out of Order" sign, and leaves you drooling into a tea towel. A planned nap is a subtle nod to self-care – a quiet little truce between you and your immune system.

In other words, you're either the napper or the napped.

LA VIDA LOCO

How To Nap Like a Mediterranean

If you want to adopt the noble siesta without sacrificing your cultural identity, here are some tips to keep you feeling more Antonio Banderas and less Captain Mainwaring:

1. Schedule It In: Find a regular time each day, perhaps early afternoon, when you'll likely feel a dip. Tell people it's a "restorative cognitive realignment break" if you must. Nothing gets respect like four unnecessary syllables.

2. Set a Gentle Alarm: Not the one that sounds like a nuclear evacuation—something melodic and tender. You want to wake up gently, not feel like Thor's hammer has resurrected you.

3. Keep It Short: Aim for 20-30 minutes. This is enough time to reboot the system, not plunge you into a three-hour fugue where you wake up thinking it's 1987.

4. Create a Ritual: Blanket? Check. Eye mask? Optional. Cup of tea before or after? Up to you. The important thing is to make it routine. Your body, much like a stubborn dachshund, responds well to routine.

The Guilt Factor and the Cost of Not Napping

Here's what happens when you push through fatigue instead of managing it:

- You start forgetting words, like "kettle" or "my name."

- You can't focus on anything more complex than a toothpaste advert.

- Your limbs feel like they're made of damp sandbags.

- You crash nap on a radiator and wake up branded like a panini.

Pacing is not just about limiting what you do; it's about strategically resting before your body goes full Game Over. It's the difference between cruising to a stop and driving straight into a hedge.

> **Your Friend on the Sofa**
>
> <u>Embrace the Siesta, Defy the Crash</u>
>
> So what's the takeaway? Napping isn't failure. It's a strategy. It's preventative medicine. The Spaniard inside you quietly says, "Lie down, cariño, and don't be daft."
>
> Let go of the British obsession with constant productivity. Your mitochondria are on strike. Your immune system is on a gap year. Your job is to stay afloat, not become the next Alan Sugar.
>
> Treat rest like oxygen: not optional, not negotiable. Schedule it. Honour it. Enjoy it.
>
> And if anyone dares to raise an eyebrow at your 2:30 p.m. recline, tell them you're conducting a high-level longitudinal recovery protocol. Then close your eyes and nap like your life depends on it—because it just might.
>
> Sweet dreams, warrior.
>
> Congratulations. You're officially pacing—Viva la siesta.

The Boom and Bust Cycle

Ah, the boom and bust cycle. The evil twin of pacing and resting. Not, sadly, an economic theory you can toss about in meetings to sound clever, but the cruel little rollercoaster gifted to those with fluctuating conditions. One day you're flying high, replying to emails like a caffeinated wizard, and the next you're collapsed on the sofa, wondering how blinking can be so exhausting.

What *Is* the Boom and Bust Cycle?

Imagine you're a phone battery with a dodgy charger. One day, you somehow get to 80% and think, "Right! Now's the time to do everything I've not done for three weeks!" So you clean the flat, sort out your inbox, climb Mount Inbox-Zoom-call, maybe even go outside. Then the next day? Dead. Not low battery. *Dead.*

This is boom and bust. You overdo it on the rare days you feel halfway human and then spend the next few days (or weeks) curled up like a half-baked crumpet, regretting your enthusiasm.

Why It Happens (And Why It Feels So Sneakily Sensible at the Time)

When you live with unpredictable health, the temptation to cram all your living into one functional day is enormous. Who can blame you? Your health has the reliability of a Southern Rail timetable, so you grab the moment.

However, the price of that productivity often arrives via express delivery. It's not laziness; it's physics. You spent all your spoons (Google 'spoon theory' if you're confused or just mildly hungry).

Spotting the Signs You're About to Bust

1. **Everything feels urgent.** Suddenly, you MUST clear your inbox, scrub the shower, reorganise the spice rack and reply to that message from 2022.

2. **You ignore your body's polite coughs.** That niggle in your back? The ache in your legs? They're whispering, "Slow down, mate." You hear them and respond with, "Later."

3. **You start making plans.** Oh, the hubris. You feel good, so you schedule three social events, promise to run a half-marathon and offer to chair a committee. Bust is laughing already.

How to Break the Cycle (Without Becoming a Hermit)

The goal isn't to never do anything fun or productive again. It's to pace yourself like a marathon runner, not a ferret on espresso.

1. **Pre-plan Your Rest** Schedule. Rest before you need it. It sounds counterintuitive, but it's like putting the bins out before they start smelling. Your future self will thank you.

2. **The 80% Rule:** If you feel you can do 100%, stop at 80%. That last 20% is probably adrenaline and hubris talking.

3. **Activity Diaries (But Make Them Sexy)** Okay, not sexy, but at least mildly informative. Jot down what you did and how it made you feel the next day. Patterns emerge. Data wins. And it makes you feel like a scientist.

4. **Say No. And Mean It.** People will ask for things. You can say no. You are not a vending machine for favours. You're a complex human with fluctuating capacity and an excellent sense of humour.

5. **Celebrate Boundaries.** Did you say no to brunch because you knew you needed rest? You legend. Light a candle. Eat a biscuit. That's a victory.

Talking About the Cycle Without Sounding Like You're Making Excuses

It's a fine line. You want to explain your reality without sounding like you're avoiding work. Try framing it like this:

- "I plan my work around my energy levels to ensure consistency, rather than risking burnout."

- "I pace my productivity to be sustainable."

- "If I do too much in one go, I crash hard. Managing that keeps me reliable in the long run."

See? You sound positively strategic. HR would weep with pride.

Bosses, Budgets and Boom Days

If your boss is reading this (hi there), know this: boom days are not signs that we're fine. They're not cures. They're temporary leases on borrowed energy. And bust days aren't laziness; they're the invoice.

Good employers understand the long game. A supported employee is productive– maybe not at 9:00 a.m. every Monday. Flexibility is an investment in quality, not a compromise on performance.

Your Friend on the Sofa

You're Not Broken, You're Brilliant

Managing the boom and bust cycle is a skill. A proper, hard-earned, nuanced, grown-up skill. You are balancing physiology, work, expectations, and that mysterious internal barometer that says, "Actually, I need a lie-down."

And you're doing it with humour, humanity, and probably in very soft clothing. That, dear reader, is not slacking. That is surviving.

Next time you feel the boom whispering, "Go on, do it all now," smile, sip your tea, and say, "No thanks. I've got pacing to do."

You're not falling behind. You're moving forward – cleverly, cautiously, and occasionally in fluffy socks.

A Diet That Won't Bankrupt You or Make You Smell of Kale

Your gut might be acting like it's got its WiFi signal and agenda. So let's talk food — without fads.

Some common themes in Long Covid diets:

- Vitamin D: Check your levels. Supplements may help mood and immune function.

- Omega-3s: Found in oily fish and walnuts. Anti-inflammatory.

- B vitamins: Support energy metabolism.

- Magnesium: Muscle, nerve, and sleep support.

Inflammation, Fasting and the Art of Not Eating Greggs for Science.

"I'm experimenting with an anti-inflammatory diet," says the blonde botoxee in skin-tight leggings, holding a turmeric latte and looking smug.

Like many of us blessed with this overachieving immune system that just won't quit (even long after the virus has buggered off), many of us take to the google navigating the world of recovery like a confused toddler at a vegan mezze. So when I read that chronic inflammation might be behind some symptoms—fatigue, brain fog, joint pain—I thought, "Right. Let's have a crack at this. I've go the square root of sod all to lose."

What's Inflammation Got To Do With It?

Now, before you roll your eyes and mutter, "not another person blaming gluten for their chakras being misaligned," this isn't that. Real science here. Peer-reviewed, PubMed-type stuff.

Several studies have linked long COVID to persistent low-level inflammation in the body. (That's *actual* inflammation, not "I can see some puffiness under my botox, time to purge.")

Cytokines—proteins that help ramp up the immune response—have been found at elevated levels months after acute infection in some long COVID patients. These little chemical messengers are helpful in short bursts, like when you need to fight off an invader. But in the long term, they can make your body feel like it's running a low-key riot in every system. Fatigue, cognitive issues, and even postural symptoms can be linked to this immune mischief.

So—how do you calm down a riot? You take away the petrol bombs and the megaphones. Enter: the anti-inflammatory diet.

The Anti-Inflammatory Diet: Or, How I Learned to Love the Lentil

This diet involves eating like the Mediterranean grandma you never had. Loads of:

- Colourful veg (as if your plate is auditioning for Strictly)

- Oily fish (salmon, sardines, mackerel—anything that smells a bit like the sea but is too posh for fish fingers)

- Whole grains (no, white bread does *not* count, Steve)

- Nuts, seeds, olive oil

- Berries and other antioxidant-rich fruits

(For goodness' sake, if you are allergic to something like nuts, don't eat them.)

And crucially, cutting back on:

- Ultra-processed foods (I miss you, cheese & onion crisps)

- Sugary drinks (a tearful goodbye to full-fat Irn-Bru)

- Alcohol (I'll allow the odd G&T, I'm not a monster)

- Caffeine

It's not a miracle cure, but it is a small thing that can be controlled in a place where very little else is. There is some evidence it works, but again, it is up to you. It makes sense to stay as healthy as possible, like an athlete training for a long run. But you are also human, and the odd treat is good for the brain.

Fasting: Or, Hangry, But Hopeful

Some people dabble with time-restricted eating, such as intermittent fasting or "not eating for a bit and hoping it helps."

Fasting apps are available, some for free, and they provide time windows for fasting, like a 14:10 window: 14 hours of fasting and 10 hours of eating. Basically, no breakfast.

Why? Some studies suggest that fasting reduces inflammation and improves mitochondrial function. That's fancy speak for "gives your cells a bit of a reset," which is appealing when your energy system feels like it's been powered by two AA batteries since 2020.

Importantly, fasting isn't for everyone. If you have any history of disordered eating, low blood sugar, or you love toast, skip this one. Truly. There are other ways to support recovery without becoming a monk who drinks black coffee at 11 am and talks about autophagy.

If That Sounds Awful.....

Suppose the idea of cutting back on your beloved biscuits fills you with despair; fear not. There are other evidence-backed approaches:

1. **Low-Histamine Diet** – Some long COVID patients report improvements on a low-histamine plan. It's fiddly, but it might help if you're having a lot of food-triggered symptoms like rashes, palpitations, or sinus congestion.

2. **Balanced Blood Sugar Diet**—Avoiding huge sugar spikes can help prevent energy crashes. Think fibre, protein, and slow-release carbs. (This is also known as "not eating cake for lunch," alas.)

3. **Anti-Processed Food Movement**—Focus on whole foods where you can. You don't need to go full Gwyneth. Even replacing one microwave curry with a home-cooked veggie

stew counts.

4. **Dietitian Support**—If you can access one, a proper dietitian (preferably one who doesn't sell supplements with their face on them) is a goldmine, especially if you're dealing with food sensitivities, weight changes, or sheer overwhelm.

What Doesn't Help
- Fad detoxes
- Juice cleanses
- Miracle powders
- Anything sold by someone with "wellness" in their Instagram handle

What Might Help
- Ginger, turmeric: Mild anti-inflammatory effects
- Probiotics: If your gut's throwing a tantrum
- Plenty of water: Yes, boring. But essential.

In short, eat a balanced diet. If you are allergic to it, don't eat it. Don't bankrupt yourself at a health shop, and never trust anyone who tells you celery juice is medicinal. Sometimes, something that tastes nice and makes you happy is good for the mood, even if it means a kilo on the scales. It's okay; you've been through enough.

> **Your Friend on the Sofa**
>
> I'm not your GP. I'm not even qualified to water your plants. But I *am* a fellow LoCo goblin who has tried some things, read the science, and found a bit of breathing room.
>
> The anti-inflammatory diet and gentle fasting helped me feel more in control of a chaotic situation. And that is a win.
>
> If that's not your jam, find what works for *you*. Recovery is not a one-size-fits-all pair of elasticated trousers. Just be kind to yourself. And maybe eat a blueberry.

RESTING

The Art of Doing Nothing (Without Guilt)

Rest. It sounds so simple, so soft, so... smug. People love to tell you to rest. "Put your feet up!" they chirp. "Treat yourself to a nap!" they chirp. But when you've got Long Covid, rest is less about relaxation and more about life support. It's not indulgent. It's necessary. But oh, the guilt. The internal voice whispers, "You haven't done enough today." The texts you haven't answered. The dishes you didn't do. The career you temporarily ghosted.

Why Rest Feels Like Failure

We live in a world that worships productivity, where your value is measured in deadlines met, emails replied to, step counts, and hustle. The rest is what you earn after the work. But with chronic illness, the formula flips. Rest is the work. And it's hard, especially if you thrived on chaos, colour-coded to-do lists, and the strange satisfaction of inbox zero.

Rewiring Your Brain: From Output to Outcome

Let's try a reframe. Instead of seeing rest as doing nothing, see it as an active strategy to prevent your health from plunging into the abyss.

Think of it as:

- Maintenance mode

- System reboot

- Biological battery charging

- My colleague calls it 'Buffering'.

This is the only thing stopping your body from declaring a strike. Your mitochondria have unionised. They demand duvet days. Listen to them.

Permission Slip: You Are Allowed to Rest

Here.

> *"I, [Insert your name], officially grant myself the right to:*
> *Lie down whenever I need to.*
> *Nap in the middle of the day without explanation.*
> *Decline social invitations with zero guilt.*
> *Watch seven episodes of a show and remember none of it.*
> *Do nothing. And still be worthy."*
> *Signed,*
> *Your Sensible Inner Voice*

Your Friend on the Sofa

<u>Resting vs. Failing</u>

You are not lazy. You are not weak. You are not giving up. You are responding wisely to your body's signals. You are choosing longevity over burnout. You are doing what works, not what looks good on LinkedIn.

And if you still feel twitchy, try this:

- Make a "reverse to-do list": write down what you did, even if it's "sat up for 10 minutes."

- Celebrate tiny wins.

- Remind yourself: you're not resting for fun. You're resting for function.

- "Chronic Illness Life Hacks"

When your body runs on fumes, anything that makes life easier deserves a Nobel Prize. These aren't just tips — they're acts of rebellion against a world designed for the bouncy and brisk.

Energy Conservation

Cooking

Slow Cooker = Best Mate: Chuck things in, press a button, and feel smug while horizontal.

Air Fryer = cheap and quick. You can cook when hungry and eat before you lose your appetite. Batch Cook on a Good Day: Freeze portions so future-you has options beyond toast.

Gadgets

Electric blankets and heated throws: Especially helpful when your circulation is in witness protection.

Shopping

Shopping Delivery pass: Do it. You will never regret not lugging a loo roll through the high street. Many delivery drivers are marvellous people, and if you need help, ask. (Some kindly supermarkets even have a notes section on the delivery details where you can leave instructions like "A bit slow getting to the door" or "Might need some help......".)

Personal Hygiene (with Dignity Intact)
- Dry shampoo: Not just for festivals anymore.

- Face wipes and no-rinse body cleansers: Great for days when showers feel like triathlons.

- Shower stool: Not glamorous. Life-changing.T

- oothbrush with timer and pressure sensor: Helps when brain fog turns brushing into a mystery.

Dressing in Clothes That Don't Make You Cry
- Elasticated waistbands: Whoever invented joggers is a genius—bonus points for the ones with pockets.

- Layerable items: When your body temperature is on a mood swing.

- Compression socks: Ugly but effective. Treat them like medical tights.

- Soft bras or no bras: There. We said it, let the girls roam free.

Mental Survival – More Gadgets
- Noise-cancelling headphones: For managing sensory overload and blocking out unsolicited advice.

- Screen dimmers and blue light filters: For the doom-scrolling you'll inevitably do.

- Notebook by the bed: Write down dreams, reminders, and grocery lists. Possibly all at once.

Admin Hacks

- Repeat prescriptions on automatic: Fewer phone calls = less rage. The Hey Pharmacy App is free and can remind you when to order and when your meds are ready to collect.

- Use a calendar app for Appointments, meds, and when you last changed the sheets.

- Set up email filters: In the future, you will weep with gratitude.

FINDING NEW JOY: WRITING, READING, MAKING STUFF (BADLY, BRILLIANTLY, OR JUST BECAUSE)

Let's be honest: Long COVID can rip through your old routines like a toddler with a glitter bomb. Maybe you used to run marathons, dance 'til dawn, or casually do yoga in ways that now feel like Olympic-level aspirations. Now, simply showering might qualify as a full-day event. But here's the truth: **joy, creativity, and stimulation don't need to be high-impact to be deeply meaningful.**

You may not have your old energy, but you still have a curious, capable mind. You still have stories, humour, imagination, and the right to *play*. Hobbies might sound fluffy or optional, but they're not

— they are **anchors. Tiny acts of defiance** against monotony. And sometimes, **the only thing keeping your brain from falling into the existential void.**

So let's reframe hobbies not as "cute distractions," but as a way to reclaim a sliver of identity in the midst of chaos.

But What Can You Actually *Do*?

You don't need to be "good" at any of this. You don't need to finish things. You don't even need to do them consistently. The goal is pleasure, not productivity. This isn't hustle culture — this is healing culture.

Here are some entry points for low-energy creativity:

- Writing – if you have more to say, or think this book is awful, write your own! Although I will warn you, editing is nightmare with brain-fog.

- Journaling: rant, reflect, write about your symptoms or what your cat thinks of your new limp.

- Flash fiction: 100 words of weirdness. No pressure. No rules.

- Poetry: Haikus, angry limericks, quiet metaphors. Therapy in syllables.

- Letter writing: to friends, to strangers, to your future self.

Reading (or Listening)

- Audiobooks are your new best friend. No eye strain, no effort.

- Podcasts: comedy, storytelling, true crime, science — something that *isn't* about viruses.

- Comic books and graphic novels: Low effort, high reward.

- Fanfiction: go deep, go weird, go joyful. No judgment here.

Making Things (Slowly, While Sitting Down, With Snacks)

- Painting, sketching, collage — even if it's just shapes and colours.

- Crochet, knitting, embroidery — repetitive, meditative, soothing.

- Baking: half batch. Or no batch. Just decorate pre-made biscuits with googly eyes.

- DIY crafts, clay, beading — or building miniature houses for imaginary mice.

Games, Puzzles, Play

- Cozy video games (Merge something, Animal Crossing, unpacking simulators).

- Word puzzles or logic games — in short, snack-sized bits.

- Board games with friends or solo — because yes, there are solo board games.

- Dungeons & Dragons — even if you're too tired to move, you can still be a wizard.

Weird & Wonderful Side-Quests
- Birdwatching (from your window counts).
- Watching competitive marble racing on YouTube.
- Making Spotify playlists with oddly specific vibes ("songs for pacing slowly in a bathrobe").
- Learning weird facts (Did you know octopuses have nine brains?)

Important Note: Be Sh*t At It.
Please don't let perfectionism or productivity guilt sneak in. This isn't about becoming an expert. It's about having *something to look forward to*. A thing that's **just yours**, that doesn't require you to be healthy, fast, smart, useful, or employed. You are allowed to make terrible art. You are allowed to abandon projects. You are allowed to do weird things that only make sense to you.

There is no prize for being the best knitter, but there is deep, feral joy in making a woollen scarf that looks like it was attacked by squirrels and still wearing it proudly.

When It Feels Like Too Much
Some days, even hobbies feel impossible. That's okay. Rest is not laziness. **Lying in bed daydreaming counts as a creative act.** Listening to one chapter of a book counts. Watching six hours of niche YouTube content counts. You're still a human being engaging with the world — at your own pace. This whole book was planned on the sofa during a horrible symptom flare. Most was dictated onto an app

and when better it was typed. It's probably not perfect, but that's not the point.

Even noticing what *might* interest you someday is enough. Curiosity is the first step.

> **Your Friend on the Sofa**
>
> Your hobby doesn't need to become a side hustle. It doesn't need to fix you. It just needs to **remind you that you're still here**. Still curious. Still worthy of joy. Even if it's small, even if it's quiet, even if it's just once a week. These are more than hobbies. These are **lifelines, breadcrumbs back to yourself**.
>
> Now go knit a jumper for an octopus. He's cold. And he's very judgy.

MAKING PEACE WITH MOBILITY AIDS

Let's talk sticks, rollators, fold-up stools, wheelchairs, and all the other things that scream "something's wrong" in public. The first time you use one? Brutal. You might cry. You might feel like you're giving up. Like you're betraying your body.

But here's the truth: Aids doesn't make you weak. It makes you mobile, and going out with someone else for the first few times helps boost confidence. My friend took me to another town where I didn't know anyone and let me have a go. She did suggest a mobility scooter until I threatened to drive it into the sea.

We all have a journey with this kind of thing. A walking stick is not a white flag. It's a bridge. It helps you go further, for longer, without crashing or falling over. It enables you to show up, allows you to live, and gives other pedestrians a warning that you might need some space.

Some people decorate theirs, give them names, or hate them. That's okay, too. Mine is called 'Walter' because I asked for my 'walking stick' and got the name wrong.

But know this: using an aid doesn't say "I can't." It says, "I'm still going on my terms."

Tips for Aids Acceptance:
- Start small: use them inside first if needed.
- Choose styles you like. Funky, floral, foldable—it's yours.
- Remind yourself: a mobility aid doesn't change who you are. It helps you be who you are.

Miscellaneous Marvels
- Reachers/grabbers: For the remote you dropped but can't be arsed to fetch.
- Bedside caddy: Keeps your snacks, meds, and Kindle from migrating into the void.
- Pill organiser: Old school, but brain fog-proof.

Your Friend on the Sofa

You are unique, and what may work for one person may not work for another. Also, timing is essential; one method may not work for you now but might later. Equally, what works now might be something you grow out of. Its evolution, you will grow, get more savvy and change. Keep trying, but always do your due diligence and check that whatever you try is from a reputable source and won't harm you.

Finding Calm in a Nervous System That Forgot How to Calm Down

So, your body's acting like it's stuck in a spin cycle. Your brain keeps buffering. Your heart races when you stand up to make a toast. And now someone's suggesting you try **mindfulness**. You might be tempted to throw a herbal tea at them.

Let's pause.

What Even *Is* Mindfulness?

In its simplest form, **mindfulness** means paying attention to what's happening now, without trying to fix it, run from it, or judge it. It's *not* the same as "thinking positively" or pretending your symptoms don't exist. It's more like saying, "Okay, this is where I am," and letting yourself be there momentarily.

Mindfulness can look like:

- Breathing slowly and noticing each inhale and exhale

- Watching clouds drift outside your window for five minutes

- Sitting with a cup of tea and *tasting it*

- Crying on the sofa and noticing how the cushion smells like crisps — and not judging yourself for either

That's it—no incense required.

But I Don't Like Mindfulness...

That's okay. Truly. Some people find it grounding, while others feel trapped in their bodies and would rather distract themselves with reality TV and beige snacks. There's **no right way** to rest your nervous system. What you are doing is distracting it.

- Not into breathwork? Try music. Sing!

- Hate silence? Try guided audio and have a good laugh at the relaxation music (usually along the lines of someone humming while trying to unblock a nostril in a cave).

- Can't sit still? Try mindful movement, such as gently rocking, stretching in bed, or slowly brushing your hair with full attention.

This is about **finding what soothes you**, not what fits a Pinterest aesthetic.

Brains Are Weird, and That's Normal

Your brain, especially post-COVID, might be on high alert 24/7. That's not a personality flaw — that's **a trauma response**, and it makes stillness feel weird or even unsafe. You're not doing it wrong if you feel more anxious during meditation. Your nervous system is just trying to protect you in clumsy ways.

Some days, you might tolerate five minutes of quiet. Other days, it's too much. Some weeks, you'll love listening to the woman on Instagram who does 'remote Reiki' because her smile is relaxing. Next week, you'll want to throw your Calm app into the sea. **This is not failure. It's flexibility.**

Woo, Optional

If breathwork, crystals, or lunar charts help you feel connected and calm, go for it. But if someone tries to tell you that your chronic illness can be healed by simply "raising your vibration," you have full permission to roll your eyes so hard you sprain an optic nerve.

You don't have to *believe* in anything mystical to benefit from simple, grounded techniques like:

- Noticing your breath

- Focusing on your senses (What can I see, hear, feel, smell?)

- Journaling about how your body feels without fixing it

- Doing *one thing* at a time, slowly

That's mindfulness, minus the sparkle filter. **Slowing Down ≠ Giving Up**

With Long Covid, rest is medicine, not laziness. But many of us struggle with this because we've been conditioned to *go-go-go*. When your nervous system won't power down, it can feel like rest is impossible, or even dangerous.

Mindfulness can help you **practice the pause**, not as a luxury, but as a survival skill. It's like saying to your body, "Hey. I know this is hard. But I'm here with you."

Some gentle ideas to try:

- **Three-breath check-in**: Pause and take three slow breaths. That's it.

- **Mindful washing**: Notice the sensation of warm water on your hands.

- **Music meditation**: Lie down and listen to one song, eyes closed.

- **Visual grounding**: Pick a colour and notice five things around you in that shade.

Final Thoughts

Mindfulness doesn't cure Long COVID. But it *can* help you:

- Rest with more ease

- Tune in to your body without panic

- Slow down enough to pace more effectively

- Notice signs of burnout before a crash

> **Your Friend on the Sofa**

And if it doesn't help today? Try something else. Or nothing at all. Just surviving with Long Covid is already enough.

Whatever you do, be kind to yourself in the process. You're not a failed yogi. You're a person with a janky nervous system trying to find peace in a body that keeps changing the rules.

So light a candle... or don't. Breathe deeply... or grumble your way through it. Either way, you're doing great.

The Bare Minimum

Survival strategies when life feels like you're running on 3% battery and someone stole the charger.

Let's be honest: when living with Long Covid, basic needs can feel like epic quests. **Eating** becomes a negotiation. **Sleeping** becomes an unpredictable lottery. And sometimes, the day's only goal is to exist semi-upright with pants on.

So let's talk about the **bare minimum** — what your body needs, what you can realistically give it, and how to meet somewhere in the middle without guilt, spreadsheets, or kale evangelists.

Food: Fuel, Not a Wellness Project

You don't need to become a nutritionist. You must **avoid starving, fainting, and, ideally, feeling worse** after eating.

Some days, food will be joy. Some days, it will be a weird, chewy obligation.

That's okay.

Realistic Tips for Feeding Your Fluctuating Body:

- **Eat what you can, when you can.** If you wake up and feel hungry, that's your moment. Don't wait. Grab something simple.

- **Keep "non-effort" foods around: crackers, yoghurt, tinned soup, smoothies, cereal, bananas, toast. If possible, make them nutrient-dense, but they should be mostly** *available.*

- **Protein matters.** Especially for healing and stabilising energy. Think: eggs, nut butter, cheese, protein bars, beans, chicken, tofu — whatever you can face.

- **Don't fear carbs.** They're not your enemy. They're brain fuel.

- **Batch or prep when you feel okay.** Got 30 minutes of energy? Make a few easy portions and shove them in the fridge or freezer. Future You will thank you with what little breath they have.

- **No shame in shortcuts.** Frozen meals? Nutritional shakes? Meal delivery? Microwaveable rice and pre-chopped veg? That's not cheating — that's strategic.

Micro-goal:
Eat something every 3–4 hours, even with a biscuit and a glass of milk. Your body's working overtime behind the scenes. Keep it fuelled.

Sleep: When Rest Isn't Restorative

Ah, yes, **the betrayal of sleep**. You lie down exhausted... and wake up just as exhausted, sometimes worse. What even is that?

Long Covid messes with the nervous system, hormones, and immune signalling — all of which can make **deep, healing sleep** frustratingly rare. But sleep *is* still worth protecting.

Strategies for Better (or Less Worse) Sleep:

- **Routine, but flexible.** Aim for similar wake/sleep times — but listen to your body. Don't panic if it varies.

- **Nap mindfully.** Naps can help, but too late in the day can cause nighttime regret. Try to keep naps short (20–60 mins), earlier rather than later.

- **Wind down.** Screens off (or at least dimmed), lights low, brain slowed. A warm bath, gentle music, or a calming audiobook can help ease the shift.

- **Don't force it.** If you can't sleep, lying there panicking rarely helps. Sit up, read something boring, try again later.

- **Try the basics: magnesium, warm drinks, weighted blankets, and cooling pillows. Explore gently. What works now might not work later,** and vice versa.

- **Ditch the guilt.** Can't sleep until 3 a.m.? Slept till noon? Your body's doing its weird thing. This is not laziness. This is healing. Let the routine be kind, not a cage.

Micro-goal:
Prioritise rest, even when sleep isn't happening. There are no demands when your eyes are closed, and low stimulation still helps.

The Bare Minimum: Survival Mode is Still Living

Some days, you'll manage food, sleep, a slow shower, and a cup of tea with your eyes open. Other days? Maybe just the tea. Perhaps not even that.

Let that be okay.

When your body is in **crash mode**, you are not "doing nothing" — you are managing a full-time, invisible workload called **existing with chronic illness**.

The Bare Minimum Might Look Like:

- Drinking water from a bottle by your bed

- Eating cold toast and calling it brunch

- Brushing your teeth lying down

- Messaging one friend to say "Still here."

- Watching three hours of YouTube while horizontal

- Not replying to anything and not apologising for it

You're still here. That counts.

> **Your Friend on the Sofa**
>
> <u>You Are Not Lazy</u>
>
> Meeting basic needs is **not basic** when your body is malfunctioning.
>
> If all you did today was nibble a cracker, lie in bed, and breathe through the fog, **you are not failing**. You are *persisting*. And persistence, even in sweatpants, is a form of power.
>
> You don't need to be productive. You don't need to optimise your healing. You need to stay. Keep going. Feed yourself. Rest. Repeat.

Making Your Home Loco-Friendly (Without Redesigning It Like a Hospital)

There's a fine line between comfort and clinical. You want a space that supports your needs but doesn't make guests ask if you're recovering from hip surgery. You want cosiness, not corridors. You want function, not fluorescent. Here's how to make your home work for your energy, pain, and fatigue — and still feel like home.

Bedroom: The Command Centre
- Invest in bedding: Soft, breathable, easy to wash. You'll be spending time here.

- Pillow pile: For propping up, reading, and the occasional existential sob.

- Bedside essentials: Lamp with a dimmer

- Reacher/grabber

- Water bottle with a straw (because the distress of being unable to sit up is greatly exacerbated by orange squash up the nose)

- Meds caddy (bonus points for labels). Snacks. Obviously.

Bathroom: The Personal Spa
- Shower stool + handheld shower: Your ticket to upright hygiene.

- Non-slip mats: Essential if you enjoy not face-planting.

- Towel robe: Towel and garment in one = genius.

- Over-toilet rails or supports: Invisible to guests. Lifesaving for you.

Living Room: Your New Office / Canteen / Therapy Den
- Blanket layering: For temperature swings. Bonus: looks decorative.

- Soft lighting: Salt lamps, fairy lights, side lamps.

- Ottomans and storage stools: Rest your feet. Hide your mess.

- Rolling trolleys: These are for medications, books, and chargers. You can push them from room to room like your own butler cart.

Kitchen: Keep It Lazy-Friendly

- Perch stools: So you can sit while pretending to cook.

- Drawer dividers: Save time hunting for forks. Nobody needs a 12-spoon chase.

- Keep snacks within arm's reach: Labelled drawers = a miracle on foggy days.

- Slow cooker, air fryer, and kettle you love: Holy trinity of energy-efficient food.

General Tips

- Hooks by doors: For bags, keys, masks. Brain fog-proofing at its finest.

- Designate a "crash zone": Somewhere comfy, quiet, soft, and non-judgmental.

- Bluetooth plugs: Turn off lights without leaving bed—Marvel at your wizardry.

Decor That Doesn't Betray You

- Art you love (distracts from your inner chaos)

- Plants that thrive on neglect

- Noise machine or white noise app

- "Please don't ring bell" sign for delivery folks (written in Comic Sans if passive-aggressive joy is your thing)

- Anything that makes you laugh or smile.

Part Six - Summary for the Foggy.

- **Pacing = doing just enough, not more.** Save spoons, avoid crashes.

- **Energy envelope = your daily limit.** Blow it = three days in bed.

- **Breathwork helps.** Belly breathe. Blow bubbles. Don't overthink it.

- **Heart rate monitoring** = stay under the crash zone. Apps help.

- **Planned naps = good.** Crash naps = drool and despair.

- **Food = fuel.** Please keep it simple. Protein + carbs = power. Kale optional.

- **Sleep = weird but still worth chasing.** Rest even if sleep fails.

- **Life hacks save energy.** Stools, gadgets, stretchy pants =victory.

- **Mobility aids = freedom, not failure.** Use them proudly.

- **Mindfulness = awareness, not incense.** Try what works. Skip what doesn't.

"You know what's worse than Long COVID?

The people who say 'just be positive!'

Sweetie, if positivity cured chronic illness, I'd be a unicorn by now."

Part Seven - WTF About the Future?

Navigating Healthcare Post Diagnosis

A Timeline of Misdiagnoses

If Long Covid had a spirit animal, it would be a chameleon that changes shape every time a medical professional walks in. What starts as "mild post-viral symptoms" quickly becomes a round-the-houses tour of UK healthcare with detours into disbelief, armchair psychology, and the ancient ritual of "try paracetamol and rest." Here is an unofficial, entirely relatable (and worryingly familiar) timeline of being misdiagnosed, underdiagnosed, or told to drink more water.

The Absurd Timeline of Trying to Get Help(Or: How to Become a Medical Mystery with a Loyalty Card for Your Local Surgery)

Week 1: The "You've Had Covid But You're Young and Healthy" Phase

You're knackered but expect to bounce back. You would mention it to your GP, but you have been on hold for an hour, and the online e-consult form closed at 8.35 am. You're getting over COVID and later fall asleep on the toilet.

Week 3: The "It's Just Anxiety" Stage
You try to call your GP again as you can't breathe walking up stairs. Because it's breathing and the GP tends to get a bit stressed about heart and breathing stuff, you get a call. GP suggests it's anxiety and normal 'getting over Covid stuff'. You nod politely while mentally drafting your autobiography: 'Breathless but Not Panicking'. The GP writes a note about an anxious patient while wondering if the fact that they haven't had a decent night's sleep since the start of the pandemic means they are likely to have a stroke on the way to Tesco. They've told you to contact them in 12 weeks if this continues and goes back to Mrs Smith's rancid toenail.

Week 6: The "Have You Tried Yoga?" Pit Stop
You're still tired. You mention joint pain to a work colleague. They recommend stretching, yoga, and possibly chamomile tea. Auntie Dorcas is 95, and she got COVID last week and is now tooling up to climb Everest. You try to imagine explaining this to your boss, who doesn't know what to think now.

Week 10: The "Could Be Anaemia, Could Be Hormones, Could Be Ghosts" Phase
You are still broken and napping like a hibernating bear. Google has told you to eat more leafy greens. Your fridge now contains three bags of spinach and a growing despair. You haven't managed to shower

standing up yet, but you bought a perching kitchen stool. Makeup has a thin layer of dust on it, and you haven't washed your hair in a week.

Month 3: The "We're Referring You Somewhere" Milestone

Bang on the 12 weeks, you have called your GP surgery. You fell asleep 3 times while on hold, and when reception asks you to describe the problem, you mutter about breathing and a pounding heart; they tell you to go straight to A&E. You book a taxi and drag yourself through the door, before dragging yourself back out six hours later with a series of ECG stickers on your chest and back, which you will find over the next two weeks. Everything was 'normal', and you will start to hate hearing that word because you know it's not.

Month 6: The "You've Been Diagnosed with Something That Isn't Real to Everyone Else" Era

You're finally diagnosed with Long Covid, maybe POTS or ME/CFS. You have known for months, but it took everyone else 5 months to catch on. Your family responds with, "Is that even a real thing?" You scream into your pillow. You are referred to a 'Long COVID Clinic', which will contact you in 6 months (because, who could have predicted, there are so many people with this diagnosis).

Month 9: The "Alternative Therapies Seem Weirdly Appealing" Chapter

You've now considered:

- Acupuncture

- Reiki

- Cold water therapy

- Hyperbaric therapy and have considered contacting the local hospital pretending you have the bends.

- Lying on the floor and hoping the Earth recharges you.

- Wearing a potato around your neck

- You draw the line at urine therapy…Just.

Month 12: The "Hyper-Researcher" Awakening

You have started with the Long COVID Clinic. They are lovely, but they can't do anything about Long COVID per se. What they can do is help you with how you feel about it. You scream into a pillow every time they mention 'acceptance'. You've become a citizen scientist. You know your HRV, BP, and CPET better than some doctors. You have spreadsheets. Your walls are covered in Post-its. You dream in PubMed.

Month 18: The "Let's Try Again" Loop

Symptoms evolve. You go back to your GP, who says, "Oh! You again." New tests. New waitlists. You now carry a tote bag full of symptom diaries, research papers, and righteous indignation. You have tried anything, including wearing a potato around your neck. Your GP cannot help with any clinical input as the BNF (British National Formulary – a book which tells you what medication can be given for what condition) doesn't have anything for Long Covid as it is 'too new'. There is something from the NHS, but it's mental health-based therapy and the odd bit of symptom management. You buy a walking stick with flowers to stop falling over in Asda. But you have discovered 'pacing', from those who have gone before with ME.

Year 2: The Enlightenment (Also Known as "Nothing Helps but Rest and Snacks")

You know your limits, pace like a pro, and stop trying to prove anything to anyone. Your diagnosis is still met with scepticism, but you no longer care and have wicked responses to the dumber questions.

Year 3: The "I'm Basically a Specialist Now" Chapter

You've amassed enough knowledge to qualify for a PhD in post-viral weirdness. You've taught junior doctors about dysautonomia in the waiting room. You have laminated diagrams. Your partner knows the difference between heart rate variability and a panic attack. At parties (if you go), you correct people who say "just tired."

Year 4: The "Acceptance With Sass" Epoch

You've stopped looking for a quick fix. Instead, you have dyed your hair neon yellow, employ the middle finger liberally, have pimped out your mobility aid with spikes and hoard the small things: moments of energy, a good day, someone who says, "I believe you." You have a hierarchy of bad advice, with "Have you tried being positive?" at the top. You own three hot water bottles, two mobility aids, a sense of humour sharper than ever and a bag of things to throw at people who suggest yoga. You're not cured. But you've evolved — like a Pokémon with a pulse oximeter. You've become resilient, resourceful, and unhinged to survive a system that wasn't built with you in mind. You pace like a pro. You've stopped trying to prove anything to anyone. Your diagnosis is still met with scepticism, but you no longer care.

You've mastered:
- Saying "no" without guilt

- Laughing at medical letters

- Explaining complex biochemistry with sock metaphors

> **Your Friend on the Sofa**
>
> You have earned your stripes. And next time someone asks if you've "tried just being more positive," you'll smile sweetly and hand them this book. They won't know what hit them, particularly if you throw it at them (do not throw it at them).

GETTING HELP (WITHOUT CRYING) ON A GOVERNMENT HELPLINE

Medical, Social, and Voluntary Services When You're Too Tired to Argue with a Phone Tree

Congratulations! You've survived a global pandemic, developed a baffling chronic illness, and are now trying to get support from a system that was confusing **before** your brain turned to mashed potatoes. Truly, you are a marvel of perseverance. Or possibly just stubborn. Either way, you're here. And now we need to get you some help.

This chapter is your survival guide to **navigating healthcare, social care, and the charming Kafkaesque jungle of paperwork** that stands between you and the support you need to function.

Spoiler: It shouldn't be this hard. But it is. So let's break it down.

Step 1: Talking to Your GP Without Screaming Into a Cushion

Your GP is the front door to all the good stuff: referrals, sick notes, support services, sometimes actual medical help. Unfortunately, the door is occasionally locked, slightly on fire, or manned by someone who thinks Long Covid is "just tiredness" and suggests drinking more water.

What to Say (When You Remember Words)

- "I have Long Covid and I need help with…"

- "I need a referral to the Long Covid clinic or relevant specialists."

- "I'd like this recorded in my notes — and also, could I have a sick note, please? Preferably one that doesn't expire in 48 hours."

Bonus Tools for the Foggy-Brained:

- A **symptom diary** — bullet points are fine. "I cried brushing my teeth" counts.

- A friend, partner, or random houseplant who can speak on your behalf when you forget what day it is

- A low voice and the quiet confidence of someone who's read the NICE guidelines at 3 am

And if they dismiss you? Ask them (gently) to put that in writing. Watch them backpedal faster than a raccoon stealing a sandwich.

Step 2: Long Covid Clinics – Yes, They Exist (Kind Of)

If your GP doesn't immediately refer you, ask, **"What Long Covid pathway is available in this area?"** Some areas have dedicated clinics. Others are still pretending COVID ended in 2022 and everyone's fine now.

Referrals may lead to:

- **Multidisciplinary Long Covid clinics** (the dream)

- **Specialists**: respiratory, neurology, cardiology, psych (less dreamy but still helpful)

- **Fatigue & rehab services** (they often have tea and understanding)

If you're told **"We don't have a clinic,"** ask for the closest alternative. If that fails, consider scribbling "LONG COVID IS REAL" in chalk outside the GP's window. Therapeutic, if not productive.

What You'll Need:

- Medical evidence (a.k.a. proof that you didn't just fancy a four-month nap)

- Descriptions of what you **can't do** reliably, safely, or consistently

- Emotional support and biscuits

Pro Tip: Don't fill in benefit forms alone unless you want to lose the will to live. Get help from:

- **Citizens Advice**

- **Disability Rights UK**

- **A very organised friend with a spreadsheet fetish**

Step 3: Social Care – Or, Help, My Sock Drawer Is More Functional Than I Am

Yes, you can ask for help around the house. No, you don't have to be 85 with a hip fracture.

Contact your local council's **Adult Social Care team** and ask for a **Needs Assessment**. This might get you:

- Help with washing, dressing, cooking, and cleaning

- Equipment (shower stools, grab rails, dignity-saving toilet gadgets)

- An **Occupational Therapist** (aka the person who might understand pacing)

Also, ask about a **Carer's Assessment** if someone else is quietly keeping your life running while you lie under a duvet of despair.

Step 4: Voluntary Help – The Kindness of Strangers (and Facebook Groups)

If the system fails you (and let's be honest, it might), there's a whole underworld of unpaid heroes keeping people like us afloat.

Look for:

- **Long Covid Support Group UK**: Massive, supportive Facebook group with info and humour

- **Long Covid Kids** (if you're parenting through the sludge)

- **Local COVID recovery groups**: Often more useful than official clinics

- **Community charities**: Age UK, Scope, Mind, local food

banks, religious organisations – many help regardless of age or background

These folks might offer:
- Food or medication deliveries
- Grants or emergency funds
- Advocacy (someone to speak for you so you don't have to cry at the council again)

And honestly? Sometimes, just hearing "I get it" from another person is the most helpful thing.

The Bare Minimum Checklist (for When You Can't Even)

If all this feels like too much (understandable), here's the **absolute basics** to try, in whatever order your brain allows:

1. **Write down your symptoms** (no poetry needed – just facts)
2. **Call your GP** and say, "I have Long Covid and I need help"
3. **Ask the council** for a "Needs Assessment"
4. **Check Citizens Advice** for benefit help
5. **Join an online support group** (just read at first if that's all you can manage)

And if all you did today was Google "how do I ask for help without crying," then you are **already succeeding.**

Your Friend on the Sofa

You Deserve Help

You are not lazy. You are not weak. You are navigating a serious condition that messes with your brain, body, and energy — and doing it in a world that still thinks a bath and a brisk walk should fix everything.

Asking for help doesn't make you dramatic. Needing support doesn't make you a failure. It makes you **a human being** who got hit by a virus and is still standing. (Or lying down. That counts too.)

So chase that paperwork in your own time. Ask for help. And if someone offers to fill in a form for you, say yes and offer them biscuits.

You are not alone in this slog. And the support? It's out there. Sometimes, just hidden behind a thousand clicks and a receptionist called Brenda.

Go gently. And don't do it all at once. You've got time — and now, a little backup.

Medication, Magic Pills...

Let's talk medication because we all hope for a magic pill and this can be the place hope goes to die.

When it comes to **Long Covid**, medication is a murky swamp full of **vague science**, **social media** witchcraft, and **doctors squinting thoughtfully while typing into Google** like you haven't just waited six months for this appointment.

Here's the honest truth:

We don't really know what works yet.

The British National Formulary (BNF) and the Scroll of Mild Disappointment

The BNF, Britain's Big Book of Meds™, is where clinicians go to check what's safe, effective, and vaguely legal. It's like menu of what can be prescribed and what for. Any medication in the book can be prescribed but if Long Covid is not on the list of permitted illnesses next to that drug it is called 'Off Label' and many Drs won't prescribe it. When it comes to Long Covid, it's all a bit... underwhelming.

Most of the advice is about **treating individual symptoms** — fatigue, breathlessness, pain, brain fog — rather than the actual condition itself. It's a bit like trying to put out a house fire with a water pistol, while someone says, "At least the upstairs bathroom seems fine."

So what do people do when mainstream medicine shrugs politely and offers a leaflet?

They turn to the Internet.

Oh, the Internet.

Welcome to the Wild West (of Wellness TikTok)

Social media is full of well-meaning people saying, "This worked for me!"

And to be fair — it might have. And to be even fairer, there are some absolute heroes out there.

But anecdote is not evidence, and **just because Annabelle from Reddit took powdered lichen extract and now runs marathons doesn't mean it will work for you.** Or anyone. Or even Annabelle, she might be lying, bright green, in a ditch somewhere.

Let's look at some of the more common "treatments" making the rounds. Again, this is not a recommendation for anything, this is an honest look and appraisal of the evidence.

1. NMN (Nicotinamide Mononucleotide)

What is it? A supplement said to boost NAD+ in the body, which in turn allegedly helps with energy production and cell repair. Popular in the "biohacking" scene, where men with podcasts take 70 pills a day and call it wellness.

What's the theory? Long Covid may involve mitochondrial dysfunction (fancy word for cells running like a knackered old blender). NMN supposedly helps your cells recharge.

What's the evidence?

- Very limited in humans.

- Some promising animal data, but you are, regrettably, not a mouse.

- Anecdotal reports vary wildly: "It saved my life!" vs. "It made me   feel like I'd licked a battery."

Should you try it?

Maybe — if you're working with a doctor or specialist and you're not allergic to hope or disappointment. But know it's **expensive**, and **not magic**.

2. LDN (Low-Dose Naltrexone)

What is it? Originally used to treat opioid addiction in high doses, in small doses it's being studied for chronic pain, fatigue, and autoimmune-type issues.

What's the theory? It may help modulate the immune system and reduce inflammation, which is suspected to play a role in Long Covid.

What's the evidence?

- Some small studies in ME/CFS and fibromyalgia show modest benefits.

- Clinical trials are ongoing for Long Covid.

- Side effects are usually mild, but start low and go slow (also great life advice generally).

Should you try it?

Possibly, if prescribed by a knowledgeable clinician. It's not a cure, but some people report small improvements in fatigue and pain. Just don't expect to leap out of bed singing show tunes.

3. Antihistamines(H1 and H2 blockers)

What is it? Over-the-counter allergy meds like cetirizine or famotidine.

What's the theory? Some Long Covid symptoms may be linked to mast cell activation —basically your immune system throwing tantrums and misfiring like a moody teenager.

What's the evidence?

- Anecdotal reports suggest it helps some people, especially with rashes, dizziness, GI issues.

- Scientific evidence is patchy but growing.

- Low risk if used appropriately — but always check with a doc, especially if combining meds.

Should you try it?

Low-cost, low-risk, may be worth a go — but it's trial and error. Do not, I repeat, do **not**, start taking antihistamines like it's a party drug. Follow the instructions and make sure your GP knows.

4. Pacing +Fluids + Salt = The Holy Trinity

What is it? Free. Glorious. Almost always annoying to hear about.

Why it matters:

- Pacing (energy management) is **the cornerstone** of many Long Covid recovery strategies.

- Salt and fluids can help with symptoms like dizziness and blood pressure drops (particularly in POTS-like presentations).

- Annoyingly effective, mostly because it's boring and nobody wants to believe something so basic might help.

Evidence base?
Strong support from ME/CFS and dysautonomia research. And frankly, if it helps, we don't argue.

5. Other Honourable Mentions:
- **Vitamin D & B12**: Often low in fatigue-related illnesses. Worth testing. Deficiency can worsen symptoms, but mega-doses won't turn you into a superhero.

- **SSRIs / SNRIs**: Sometimes prescribed for brain fog, anxiety, pain. Not a sign that "it's all in your head," but that your nervous system is under siege.

- **Antivirals & Immunomodulators**: Still largely in clinical trial territory. Promising, but **not available to most people outside research settings**.

The Bottom-line (Literally)
- **There is no single cure yet.**

- The evidence base is **small**, still growing, and wildly inconsistent.

- Be wary of anyone promising you a miracle in exchange for £200 and a suspiciously unlabelled bottle of drops.

But also — keep hope. Tiny, evidence-based hope. Some things *do* help. For some people. Sometimes.

- And it's okay to try things. Just don't blame yourself if they don't work. You're not failing treatment. **The treatments are failing you.**

- Until science catches up, we're all part Guinea pig, part philosopher, part detective.

- So take your meds (or don't). Try the supplement(or don't). But always keep your scepticism in one hand and your snacks in the other.

- Because frankly, if anyone's going to discover the cure, it's probably someone on day 49 of brain fog who accidentally creates a wonder drug while mixing Berocca and jam.

- Stranger things have happened. (Like, you know... *this entire decade*.)

Is This a Treatment or a Pseudoscientific Scam?

(*A handy guide for the chronically exhausted and reasonably suspicious*)

When you're ill, desperate, and abandoned by traditional medicine's shrugging arm, anything promising relief starts to look alike a viable option. Suddenly, a man on Instagram with suspiciously white teeth and a tan that says "not NHS-approved" is telling you that bee venom and moonlight baths can "recalibrate your mitochondria."

And you're tired. And sick. And maybe—just maybe—you think, *"Can it hurt to try?"*

Yes. Yes, it can.

Let's walk through how to spot a **legit** treatment, a **harmless placebo**, and a **full-blown scam dressed as 'healing energy'**.

The Scamometer: Six Questions to Ask Yourself

1. Does it promise a cure for *everything*?

If it claims to fix fatigue, inflammation, anxiety, IBS, eczema, your mum's arthritis, AND your credit score — **run**. That's not medicine. That's multilevel marketing in a lab coat.

Legit treatments: Work for specific symptoms, sometimes mildly, sometimes inconsistently.

Scams: "This single herb will heal you entirely in 3 days, also grow back your eyebrows."

2. Is it only being sold by one person, on one weird website, and costs £129.99 for a 'starter pack'?

If the only way to get it is through a personal link, and it comes with a PDF guide written entirely in Comic Sans — **no**.

Legit treatments: Usually have a licensed provider, pharmacy access, or at least regulation.

Scams: "You can't get it on the NHS because Big Pharma doesn't want you to know." (Quick note – if you every thought a nurse was in the pay of big pharma, ask yourself why they still go to work and come home with pee in their shoes?)

3. Are there actual studies, or just testimonials from someone named Moonchild in a fringed poncho?

We love Moonchild. But unless Moonchild ran a double-blind placebo-controlled trial, **her vibes are not evidence.**

Legit treatments: May have small studies or at least trials in progress.

Scams: "Look, this guy on YouTube's aura improved dramatically after three drops of dragon oil."

4. Do they say doctors don't want you to know about it?

Ah yes, the global medical conspiracy to suppress your healing so they can keep... running overstretched clinics with broken airconditioning?

Legit treatments: Are tested and scrutinised, sometimes slowly and frustratingly. (Practicing evidence based medicine is the difference between the person eating the pretty red berry no one knows the name of and being the person who is watching to see what happens.)

Scams: "Doctors are part of the system, but I'm a healer and a carpenter and I know better."

5. Is it mostly just expensive wee?

Supplements with 42 ingredients, only three of which are even pronounceable, won't necessarily kill you — but they might make your kidneys roll their eyes.

Legit treatments: Usually have dosing, guidance, and oversight.

Scams: "This sea moss blend is infused with love and copper ions. It's £89 per spoon."

6. Are they selling hope, or selling answers?

There's a difference between hopeful experimentation and *cultish certainty*. One says, "This might help, here's some data." The other says, "Do this or stay sick forever."

Legit treatments: Leave space for uncertainty.

Scams: "You just didn't do it right. That's why it didn't work. Try again — also buy the gold version."

Red Flag Phrases to Watch Out For

- "Suppressed by the mainstream medical establishment"

- "Quantum healing frequencies"

- "Just detox harder"

- "Raise your vibration"

- "No side effects – because it's natural!" (Can I remind you Hemlock is natural)

- "Western medicine only treats the symptoms, not the cause (which is trauma from Atlantis)"

So... Can You Try It Anyway?

Here's the honest bit:
You're allowed to try weird things.
Just do it **safely** and **informed**.

Ask:

- Can I afford this without skipping groceries?

- Is this backed by *any* science?

- Am I replacing something useful with something shiny?

- Is this making me feel in control, or just giving me false hope?

If you're working with a clinician, talk to them. If you're not (because the system is failing you), try to be your own gentle sceptic.

And remember: if something works for you, even if it's placebo — that's still valid. Just don't let anyone convince you that *they* are your only path to healing.

Especially if they call themselves "Doctor" but spell it "Docturr."

Relationships, Work and the Real World

When Friends Disappear – How to Talk to People Without Screaming 'I'M ILL, NOT LAZY'

There's nothing quite like telling someone you've got Long Covid and watching their eyes glaze over as they prepare to say to you about their cousin's ex who cured it with goat yoga.

The Problem with Invisible Illnesses

People like tidy narratives. You were ill, and you got better—end of story. But Long Covid laughs in the face of linear recovery. Some days you're fine-ish. Other days, you're horizontal. It's hard to explain without sounding like you're exaggerating or seeking attention.

The Art of the Script

Sometimes it helps to have pre-prepared phrases. Here are a few:
"I'm managing a post-viral condition that affects my energy levels. It's

unpredictable." "I'd love to, but I must pace myself now." "It's not that I don't want to come. If I do, I might not function for three days." "I look fine, but that's because you're not seeing me when I collapse on the bathroom floor."

Humour as Armour

Joking about it can make it easier for you and them. "My immune system threw a tantrum and never stopped. "I'm on the long-haul Covid express. No stops, no refunds. "Today's symptoms brought to you by the number 7 and the letter D for 'debilitating'."

Solidarity: Find Your People

Join support groups, follow advocates online, and vent anonymously or loudly, depending on your preference. Knowing you're not alone makes a huge difference. You are not the only one cancelling dinner plans for the fifth time.

When to Ghost People (Kidding… Mostly)

If someone repeatedly doesn't get it, doesn't try, and makes you feel worse about yourself, it's okay to create distance. Chronic illness is exhausting enough without managing other people's ignorance. You don't owe anyone an explanation. Just because your illness isn't visible doesn't mean it isn't real.

Also, some people get in a chronically sick mindset. They become all about sickness, and sometimes that can sap hope and positivity. You do not owe anyone else with Long Covid at the expense of anything which makes your life worth living. If today is not the day for this, or you need to distance yourself, remember you are on different journeys, and maybe they will converge later.

You can let go with love and move on.

"How Are You Today/Now?" – The Daily Dilemma

Few questions in life are as loaded, deceptively complex, and existentially exhausting as *"How are you?"*

It's supposed to be simple. Casual. A social nicety that can be volleyed back and forth like a polite game of tennis.

But when you're living with Long COVID – or any chronic illness – that question becomes a minefield. Do you answer truthfully and risk being seen as a walking medical file? Do you smile and say, *"Fine, thanks!"* while actively wondering if you have enough energy to make it to the toilet later?

It's a decision we make countless times, often on autopilot. But the emotional arithmetic behind it? Exhausting.

Option A: The Classic British Lie – "I'm Fine"

The default answer. The lie that oils the wheels of small talk.

"I'm fine" is safe. It avoids awkward silences, pitying looks, or worse, unsolicited advice about turmeric.

You might choose this option because:

- You're tired of explaining.

- You don't want to be *that person*.

- You're trying to feel normal, if only for a moment.

- You can't be bothered to support someone through your illness again emotionally.

Sometimes, minimising feels like a mercy. You get to skip the winces and the worried eyebrows. You get to have a conversation about literally anything else.

And yet...

Option B: The Honest Answer – "Actually, Not Great"

Sometimes, the truth comes out. Maybe you're too tired to filter. Perhaps the person asking feels safe. Maybe you're just fed up with pretending.

You answer honestly:

- "Today's tough."

- "I'm flaring pretty badly."

- "Everything hurts, and I think my legs are made of soup."

And then... the awkward pause.

The well-meaning "Oh no!" or "But you look great!" or "Have you tried yoga?"

Being honest is brave. But it can also feel risky. You worry you'll become defined by your illness. That people will avoid you. That you've killed the mood.

So you choose carefully, every time. You weigh your honesty like it's a currency.

The Identity Trap

The tricky bit is this: when you've been sick for a long time, being sick starts to become part of your identity—not because you want it to, but because it's always there. It shapes your days, limits your choices, and is the lens through which you move through the world.

So when someone says, *"How are you?"* it can feel like they're asking: "Who are you today?"

And sometimes you want to scream, *"I am not just this illness! I am still funny and sarcastic and capable of reciting entire scenes from 'The Vicar of Dibley'!"*

But other days, the illness is front and centre. It's taking up all the space.

So what do you do?

You Choose. That's the Power.

There's no rulebook for answering "How are you?" There's only your truth, boundaries, and energy levels on any given day.

You might say:

- "Honestly? It's been rough. But I'm glad to see you."

- "Do you want the short answer or the real answer?"

- "I'm still breathing and mildly caffeinated. Let's call that a win."

Or you might smile and say *"Fine"* and change the subject – not because you're hiding, but because you've decided that's all you want to give today. That's not dishonesty. That's discretion.

When Honesty Costs You

Let's talk about the tricky bit. Sometimes, when you're consistently honest about how you feel, people start to pull away.

Maybe they don't know what to say or feel helpless. Maybe your honesty reminds them that health is not guaranteed, and people don't enjoy being reminded of that.

You might lose people. That's not on you.

Some might see it as a sign of weakness, and they may prey upon that. Be mindful of what you share, with who, and what the fallout might be. Be honest if you will but, most importantly, be smart.

The friends worth keeping are the ones who can hold space for your truth without needing you to perform wellness—the ones who don't require you to be "fixed" to be still worth their time.

But I Don't Want to Be The Sick One All the Time

Totally fair. You don't want every interaction to be a recap of your symptoms. You don't want to feel like a burden, or like your illness is the only interesting thing about you.

Here's the thing: being honest doesn't mean being **only** about illness.

You can say: *"Yeah, things are hard right now. But please tell me what's going on in your world. I need a distraction from my own melodrama."*

You get to steer the conversation. You get to be complex. You get to be sick, curious, interested, fed up, and hilarious – all in one sentence.

Authenticity Doesn't Always Mean Full Disclosure

Being authentic doesn't mean you owe everyone your full medical chart. It means being *true to yourself*. That might look like:

- Choosing when and with whom to be candid.

- Protecting your energy by keeping things light.

- Being direct when you need support.

You don't have to tell your story to everyone who asks. You don't have to explain your illness at every coffee catch-up. You can say, *"I'm doing okay, but let's talk about something else today."*

Your Friend on the Sofa

<u>You Are More Than This</u>

When you're in it every day, it's easy to forget. But you are more than this illness.

You are a friend. A listener. A book lover. A sarcasm ninja. A parent. A creator. A connoisseur of particular biscuits. You are a thousand things, not just the one.

So when someone asks, *"How are you?"* answer however you need to at that moment. You are not obligated to be performatively positive, nor are you required to give them the unedited truth.

Just remember: *You still have to decide who you are today.*

Small People Who Grow Up Fast

Parenting While Knackered

Let's talk about parenting with Long Covid, "trying to keep small humans alive while you feel like a punctured beanbag." This isn't about winning at parenting. This is about surviving it with everyone mostly intact, and hopefully nobody accidentally putting the dog in the fridge.

Parenting is hard enough when you're healthy. With Long Covid, it becomes a slapstick juggling act performed from a mattress. Lowering the Bar (And Then Lowering It Again)

Your idea of parenting may have once involved wholesome craft projects, trips to the park, and carefully curated lunchboxes shaped like woodland creatures. It's about ensuring your kids are fed, semi-clothed, and haven't set fire to anything.

And that's OK.

Your child's emotional health doesn't depend on you being a Pinterest mum. It depends on being loved, seen, and occasionally supervised. Having a parent with a chronic condition might inspire them to find a cure or go into a caring profession. Ill or not, you have the same chance as everyone else of being the parent of Mother Teresa of Boris Johnson (Sorry).

Helpful Hacks:

- Declare pyjama days. No one argues with a parent in fluffy socks.

- Delegate like you're royalty. Let older kids take turns making cereal dinners.

- Batch record cartoons so you can nap without guilt.

- Invent "quiet games" like "Let's Pretend Mummy Is a Statue."

Guilt Is Inevitable, But Useless.

You'll feel guilty for missing school events. You'll feel guilty for not playing tag. You'll feel guilty for ordering takeout three days in a row.

Here's a truth bomb: the best thing you can teach your kids is empathy, boundaries, and self-care. And they learn that by watching you.

Also, nobody's kids thrive on carrot sticks and phonics workbooks alone. Screen time isn't failure. It's survival.

> **From Fellow Knackered Parents on the Sofa**
> "I keep a 'yes box' of safe snacks and activities they can access without me."

"We do bedtime story podcasts. I lie down, they listen. Win-win."

"I taught my teenager to make tea. He's now a barista-level legend."

Your Kids Will Be Okay. Children are weirdly adaptable. They don't need perfect parents. They need you, however you show up. And they'll probably grow up funnier, more resilient, and very good at making toast.

Sex, Dating, and Other Things You're Too Tired For

Let's talk about the one more draining than a full-body crash: trying to be sexy when your mitochondria are on strike.

The Libido Rollercoaster

Some people with Long COVID experience hormonal changes that affect libido. Others are too knackered to think about it. Then there's the weird combo of wanting intimacy but not having the physical capacity for it. All valid. All normal.

Communicating in Bed (Not Just the Fun Kind)

If you're in a relationship:
- Be honest. Explain how your symptoms affect intimacy. Suggest alternatives: cuddling, chatting, watching TV to-

gether.

- Remember: emotional closeness is sexy too.

If you're dating:
- Mention your condition when it feels right. If they ghost you, it's a great early warning system.

- Pace your dates. Coffee instead of clubs. Walks instead of wild nights.

- Bring snacks. Always.

- Consent Is Still Key – Being ill doesn't mean you lose autonomy. Boundaries are more critical than ever. You can stop halfway. You can say no even if you said yes last week. You don't owe anyone an explanation for not feeling up to it.

Body Image and Feeling Like a Wreck

It's hard to feel desirable when you're in pyjamas 80% of the time. But the sexiest thing is someone who listens to their body, takes care of it, and treats it with respect. Also, no one looks good under fluorescent lights, not even celebrities.

The Relationship Survival Kit

Long Covid doesn't just affect you. It affects everyone around you, especially partners, carers, and the people you live with. It turns romance into routine, intimacy into admin, and communication into a guessing game powered by brain fog.

When One Person Becomes a Nurse (And No One Asked For That)

Your partner may be picking up the slack—doing more housework, errands, or emotional labour. They might feel overwhelmed, scared, or even resentful. You might feel guilty, angry, or worried that you're dragging them down. None of that makes either of you bad people. It makes you human.

Practical Tools:

- Check-ins: A weekly "how are we doing?" chat (yes, even if it's while horizontal).

- Love languages: Speak each other's language even in small ways. If yours is acts of service, a cup of tea means the world.

- Don't fake wellness: Hiding symptoms to make your partner feel better usually backfires.

- Keeping the Spark (Sort Of) Alive- Cuddling counts. Watch shows together that require no mental effort. Leave each other silly notes or texts. Laugh together. It's medicinal.

Sex and Intimacy: A Quick Pep Talk

Desire may go into hibernation. That's OK. You can have intimacy without intercourse, connection without energy, and closeness without pressure. Communicate. Be patient. And maybe buy some ridiculously soft blankets.

Occasions and Leaving the House

The Spoonie Social Survival Guide

Birthdays: Gift early. Avoid late nights. Suggest an alternative, like brunch or a walk.

Outside events and garden parties: Choose a shade. Bring comfy seating. Skip standing in queues. Ask someone to make you a plate.

"You coming out tonight?"

Consider replying with a stock photo of a blanket and a tea mug. Or, honestly, "I'm not up to it, but have the best time and post a picture so I can live vicariously."

When You Go But Regret It Mid-Way

Locate the nearest toilet/quiet room. Say, "I'm just going to grab some air" and vanish if needed. Lie. Honestly, "Stomach" is an excuse that ends most questions.

Dealing with Guilt and FOMO

You're not being antisocial. You're energy-selective—big difference. You'll show up when you can. And when you do, you'll bring empathy, humour, and the best chat.

> **Your Friend on the Sofa**
>
> Do not stop planning and booking things because you 'probably' won't go. If you have a class, explain to the teacher that sometimes you can't come or have a friend on standby who will always use your ticket. Don't narrow your world; have a plan in your pocket.

work

One of the trickiest things about Long Covid? It's invisible. You don't look ill. There's no plaster cast or hospital bracelet. So when you tell your boss you're still struggling, they often tilt their head like a confused spaniel and say, "But you had Covid months ago, right?"

Cue: the art of the sick note, the awkward HR conversations, and the sudden urge to send your manager a link to the latest NICE guidelines.

Getting Time Off (Without Guilt or Grovelling)

You are legally entitled to sick leave. You don't need to prove your worth by logging into Zoom with a 39-degree temperature and a hot water bottle taped to your face.

Fit Notes:

You can self-certify illness for 7 days. After that, get a GP to write a fit note. Be clear: Use phrases like "post-viral fatigue," "Long Covid," and "Post-Exertional Malaise."

Occupational Health:

Ask your employer for a referral. It sounds formal, but they may be helpful.

Know Your Rights (Because Not Everyone Does)

Under the Equality Act 2010, Long Covid can be considered a disability. That means you're entitled to reasonable adjustments at work.

What counts as 'reasonable'?

- Reduced hours or phased returns.

- Home working (if your job allows it)

- Longer breaks or rest areas.

- Flexible deadlines

Useful resources:www.gov.uk/long-Covid

If your boss isn't aware of this stuff, educate gently. Maybe start with, "Would you like to read something helpful?" Be candid. Say, "I can't" Without Apologising. You are not lazy, flaky, or making it up. Saying, "I can't do that right now," isn't a personal failing. It's a boundary, and boundaries are sexy.

Remember: You are ill. You deserve support. And if your boss gives you grief, remind them of how expensive employment tribunals are.

Long Covid and Employment – Redefining Your Work Self

Let's talk about the elephant in the office: work. More specifically, trying to work like you used to while your body has quietly resigned and your brain is on a part-time contract. For many, Long Covid has forced a radical rethink of career, capacity, and identity. You're no longer the early-starting, late-finishing, deadline-eating machine you used to be. And you know what? That's not failure. That's reality. If any colleagues struggle with that, it's their issue, and maybe a quick chat with HR will close that one down.

The Myth of Bouncing Back

The post-illness fairy tale goes like this: you get sick, take some time off, rest up, then spring back to your desk with newfound gratitude and slightly better hydration habits. Long Covid does not care for that narrative. Instead, you might find yourself staring blankly at your screen, forgetting basic words, rereading the same email six times, and crying because someone asked for a Zoom catch-up.

- Changing Expectations (Of Yourself)

- You may need to:Work fewer hours.

- Shift to a slower pace.

- Take naps between meetings.

Prioritise rest like your life depends on it (because it does). This isn't slacking. It's adapting. Reframing your worth away from productivity and toward sustainability is the new power move.

Cognitive Chaos at Work

Brain fog at work is the adult equivalent of dreaming you turned up to an exam naked. You sometimes forget names, tasks, passwords, or even your job title.

Strategies:

- Use lists, alarms, post-its, and digital reminders.

- Repeat back instructions out loud. (Bonus: it makes you sound very thorough.)

- Ask for written instructions.

- Blame your "new system," not your scrambled neurons.

Disclosure Dilemmas

Do you tell your employer? If you need adjustments, yes. If you're scared of stigma, it's also valid. Pick a manager you trust. Explain symptoms, not diagnosis, if needed. Script: "I'm managing a post-viral condition that affects energy and concentration. With the right support, I can still contribute meaningfully."

When Your Career Identity Takes a Hit

Maybe you were the go-to person. The team rocks. The one who pulled all-nighters and solved crises before lunch. Now, a spreadsheet gives you vertigo and replying to an email deserves a biscuit. It's grief. Professional grief. And it's OK to mourn the version of you who did it all. But here's a secret: you're still valuable. Maybe even wiser, more bound, and empathetic—the kind of colleague who asks how people are and listens to the answer.

Discrimination, Doubt, and Dents to Your Reputation

Invisible illness invites invisible judgment. "You don't look ill." "She's always off sick." "Maybe she's not cut out for this."

If you feel your reputation is taking hits:

- Keep a work journal: track symptoms and impact.

- Be clear and consistent in communication.

- If possible, involve HR or Occupational Health to formalise adjustments.

You may have to advocate harder than seems fair. But you're not alone—and you're not making it up.

SURVIVING WORK WITH A FLUCTUATING CONDITION

Let's be honest. Working with a fluctuating condition is a bit like trying to assemble flat-pack furniture in the dark while someone reads the instructions to you in Latin. Some days you're smashing it – metaphorically, unless you work in demolition – and other days you're horizontal, wrapped in a blanket burrito, wondering if this is your new full-time job now.

People without fluctuating conditions – let's call them consistents – have the privilege of waking up and generally knowing how their bodies will behave. It's very smug of them. They bounce into caffeinated and perky meetings while you're trying to work out if your joints will support you long enough to hobble to the kettle.

So, how do you balance work and illness without going full Basil Fawlty and snapping at everyone in a glorious but career-ending meltdown?

Glad you asked.

Admit You Are Not a Cyborg

One of our first mistakes is pretending we're absolutely fine when we're about as stable as a weather app. "I'm great," we say, as we attempt to type with one hand because the other has suddenly gone on strike.

But here's the thing: you're not a malfunctioning robot. You're a person. A spectacularly knackered, occasionally brilliant, frequently horizontal person. You don't need to perform health checks just because Janet in Accounts once sprained her ankle in 2004 and "still came into work."

By the way, Janet, no one asked.

Email Autoresponders Are Your New Best Friend

You know those perky "Out of Office" messages people use when they're off in the Algarve sipping cocktails and sunburning their shoulders? Time to use them with flair.

Sample:

Hello, thanks for your email. I'm currently experiencing a spontaneous collapse of my nervous system and will respond when my brain reboots. If urgent, please scream into the void or try again later. Cheers!

You'd be surprised how understanding people become when you politely but firmly let them know you are not currently in the mood for spreadsheets.

The Art Of Pacing

You might find yourself in a situation where your energy is flatter than a pancake run over by a lorry, but you still need to appear professionally alive. Yes, sometimes you might be in a role when 'presenteeism' is seen as next to godliness. Here are a few tips:

- Zoom Meetings: Turn off your camera. You can be honest about needing to conserve your energy in a safe environment or claim internet issues in one that is not. While your coworkers argue over who muted Steve again, you can gently pass out into a bowl of cereal.

- The Email Delay Game: Again, if things are unsafe, schedule your replies to send later in the day. This creates the illusion of sustained productivity rather than one manic burst of energy at 9:03 a.m. followed by a six-hour nap. It is best to be honest, but again, the world is not perfect, and neither are energy spikes and furrows. Just bear in mind that you should never fall into 'Boom and Bust' cycles.

HR Helpful or Harrowing?

HR departments are like weather forecasters: occasionally functional, sometimes amazing, sometimes baffling, and usually ill-prepared for the storm you're bringing.

Some HR reps are delightful unicorns who will bend over backwards to accommodate you. Others will smile sweetly while asking if you're sure your diagnosis is real, because "you don't look ill." This is your cue to either:

- Politely educate them.

- Or lob your medical file at them like an Olympic discus.

Don't be afraid to request accommodations, though. Legally, you're entitled to them. This includes flexible hours, remote work, assistive tech, and – most crucially – the right to occasionally say "No, thank you, I'd rather not burst into flames today."

Meetings You Should Absolutly Cancel

There is a misconception that meetings are inherently productive. This is a lie. Most meetings are, at best, group therapy with PowerPoint. If your body has entered "Nope Mode," you are entirely within your rights to cancel with dignity.

Suggested excuses:

- "Currently engaged in a tactical negotiation with my immune system. Results pending."

- "Developing a close, horizontal relationship with my heating pad. Non-negotiable."

- "Not dead, but deeply adjacent."

If all else fails, schedule the meeting for 3:30 p.m. on a Friday. No one will attend anyway.

Co Workers – The Good, The Bad and the Alarmingly Clueless

Some colleagues will surprise you with their compassion, bringing you tea or asking what support you need. Then there will be the others – let's call them Derek. Derek doesn't mean to be offensive. He genuinely believes that yoga cures all ailments and that turmeric is a miracle, he rides a bike into work, wears the helmet up to the fourth floor and is always slightly damp.

Derek might say things like:

- "Have you tried just thinking positively?"

- "You don't seem ill to me."

- "I read an article about how cold water swimming resets your mitochondria."

Remember: it is not your job to educate Derek. But it is your right to respond with a facial expression that conveys, "If you speak again, I will unfriend you in real life."

Working From Home – Heaven or Hellscape?

Ah, the joys of remote work. No commuting, no trousers, and you can hold meetings wrapped in a heated blanket. But beware: working from home also means your boundaries can erode faster than a biscuit in tea.

Suddenly, it's 9 pm and you're still fiddling with that spreadsheet because you "had a nap earlier and now you feel guilty." Stop that. Guilt is not a productivity tool. It's a sneaky little gremlin sent by capitalism.

You are allowed to rest. Resting is part of the job when your body plays musical chairs with your energy levels.

When It All Goes Tits Up

Despite your best efforts, there will be days when it all falls apart. You miss deadlines. You forget meetings. You send an email to the CEO that reads "banana" because your brain fog was so dense it felt like you were typing underwater.

On those days, forgive yourself. Seriously. You're not weak. You're not lazy. You're a bloody legend for even trying.

And if anyone questions your work ethic, kindly point out that you've been working twice as hard to seem half as functional – and that's a mathematical miracle.

> **Your Friend on the Sofa**
>
> Managing a fluctuating condition while trying to hold down a job is like juggling flaming torches while someone occasionally sets your trousers on fire. You are doing the impossible, and you're doing it with style (or at least with slippers and a passive-aggressive mug that says "I'm silently judging you").

> Celebrate the wins – even the tiny ones. You answered two emails? Incredible. You showered before noon? Nobel-worthy. You made it through a Monday without crying or punching a printer? You're basically a superhero.
>
> Keep going. You've got this. And when you don't, that's okay too. Just blame Derek.

What If You Can't Go Back?

Some people change careers, go part-time, or stop working altogether. That can feel like failure, especially in a society that links work to worth. But your value is not tied to a payslip. You are still smart. You are still skilled. You are still you. And any employer, friend, or family member who can't see that? They're the ones missing out.

Redefine Success

Maybe success now looks like:

- Working one solid hour without a nap.

- Asking for help without guilt.

- Leaving on time, always.

- Saying "I need a break" without apologising.

> **More From Your Friend on the Sofa**
>
> Small wins count. You're navigating work on hard mode—and you deserve a trophy for every day you show up, however that looks.

You're not lazy. You're adapting. You're not less. You're learning a new way. And you're doing it while half the world still thinks "brain fog" is a cute excuse to forget meetings. Which makes you, frankly, a legend.

Part Seven - Summary for the Foggy.

- Chronic illness messes with **social norms**, friendships, work—and your sense of self.

- You're often stuck choosing between **honest answers and emotional energy**.

- People disappear, misjudge, or offer turmeric—**nonunderstanding is common**.

- Parenting, sex, and dating? **Still possible—but with pyjamas and pacing**.

- Work with Long Covid means **adjusting, advocating, and letting go of old identities**.

- You are **not lazy, not a burden, and not alone**—you're surviving a system not built for you.

> "I don't rise and shine anymore —
>   I wake up and wheeze like an old radiator trying to die with dignity."

Part EIGHT - WTF ABOUT Money?

Chronic illness doesn't just attack your body. It goes for your bank account, too.

It arrives uninvited, eats your energy, steals your career momentum, and then has the nerve to hand you a stack of receipts. Because being ill isn't just exhausting – it's expensive.

We often talk about the emotional and physical costs of long-term illness. But let's talk about the literal cost because you can't pay your rent in positive affirmations. And compassion doesn't cover the price of mobility aids or prescription co-pays.

The Financial Gut Punch

Here's how the average chronic illness journey might look financially:

1. You get sick and start missing work. You might take it if you're lucky enough to have sick leave.

2. You keep getting sick. You use up your leave. Your savings, if you had any, start shrinking.

3. You try to get help. But navigating benefits, insurance claims, or workplace adjustments feels like explaining quantum mechanics through an intercom at a broken drive-thru.

4. You start paying for things you never budgeted for: special diets, supplements, therapies, private appointments because the waiting list is now longer than your illness has lasted, equipment, travel, heating, electricity, more heating, more electricity.

Repeat for weeks, months, or years.

The Hidden Cost of Being Unwell

The financial burden of chronic illness isn't just about big, scary bills. It's also the small, relentless ones:

- Higher utility bills because you're home all day.

- Increased food costs from needing convenience or dietary-specific items.

- Transport costs from not being able to use public options.

- Clothes to accommodate changing bodies or medical devices.

- Out-of-pocket medication costs.

- Therapy (if you're trying to stay sane).

- Missed promotions, freelance gigs, or creative projects.

These things chip away at your stability – not with a bang, but with a constant, stress-inducing drip.

The Career Crunch

Jobs are tricky when you're chronically ill.

Some people lose them outright. Others are forced into reduced hours or 'voluntary' redundancies. Self-employed folks face feast-or-famine months with zero safety net. And let's not even get started on how hard it is to explain chronic illness in a job interview without sounding like a health risk with a to-do list.

Even if you can keep working, you might do so at significant personal cost. You're using up all your energy to clock in. There's nothing left over. Your job becomes your entire life, not in the fun, ambitious, I-love-my-career way. More in the "I worked 20 hours this week and now need two days in a dark room" kind of way.

The Bureaucratic Battlefield

Now for everyone's favourite nightmare: applying for financial help.

Whether it's government support, insurance payouts, or workplace accommodations, the system is often not designed with chronic illness in mind. It's intended for acute, visible, one-time conditions. Not fluctuating, invisible, "but you were fine yesterday" kinds of diseases.

You'll need:

- Endless paperwork.

- Letters from doctors who barely know your name.

- The stamina of a caffeinated goat.

- A sense of humour and/or a breakdown.

And if you're rejected? You might need to appeal, which means more paperwork. Possibly a tribunal. More emotional labour. All while you're still... you know... sick.

How To Survive

Let's be real – there's no one-size-fits-all solution. But here are some sanity-saving strategies:

1. Track Everything

You don't need a fancy spreadsheet, but having a rough idea of what's going out and why can help you spot patterns and prioritise.

Even if all you learn is, "Wow, I spend a fortune on takeaways because I can't cook," – that's helpful info. You might look for cheaper options, batch cooking on a good day, or meal delivery support schemes.

2. Know Your Rights

You may be eligible for government benefits, grants, disability support, transport discounts, or energy help. These vary by country and region, but a good place to start is:

- Disability rights organisations

- Citizens Advice (UK)

- Social workers attached to medical teams

- Online communities

3. Ask For Help

This one's hard, but sometimes your friends, family, or community want to help—they don't know how.

Maybe someone can:

- Cook a few meals

- Drive you to appointments

- Share equipment or supplies

- Help with benefit applications

Asking isn't a weakness. It's resourcefulness.

4. Work With What You've Got

Suppose you're still working or want to, investigate flexible or remote roles. Some people pivot into freelancing, creative work, or running small online shops based on their skill sets. This isn't easy, but for some, it's a way to maintain dignity, purpose, and a little bit of income on their terms.

And for those who can't work at all right now? That's valid. Rest is not laziness. Survival is a full-time job.

5. Build A Supportive Network

Find people who understand. Online forums, social media groups, and local support networks can connect you with others who get it – and who might share tips, humour, or even resources.

You're not alone in this. Not even financially.

Benefits and Bureaucratic Bingo

The UK benefits system is like trying to do an escape room blindfolded, hungover, and mid-crash, even before the recent governmental system fiddling.

This section is your torch, compass, and occasional swear jar as we wade through the nitty-gritty of getting financial help when you're too unwell to work.

Sick Notes: Your First Line of Defence

If you're employed and need time off, the first step is to get a Fit Note (formerly called a sick note) from your GP. This confirms that you're too unwell to work. We've discussed this before, but it is worth reiterating in this context.

Top Tips:
- Be specific: tell your GP exactly how Long Covid affects your day-to-day.

- Ask for "phased return" if you're trying to return gradually.

- Keep copies—your employer and any benefit agency will want them.

You're legally entitled to Statutory Sick Pay (SSP) if you're too sick to work and meet the criteria.

Statutory Sick Pay (SSP)
What is it?
- Paid by your employer for up to 28 weeks
- Currently £116.75 per week (as of 2025)
- Paid after the first 3 days of absence

Eligibility:
- You must earn at least £123/week (as of 2025)
- Be employed (not self-employed)

Apply via your employer.
- They may have their HR forms/process
- Ask for an HR contact if you're unsure

After 28 weeks? You may move to ESA.

Employment and Support Allowance (ESA)

What is it? A benefit for people who are ill or disabled and can't work. Two main types:

- **New Style ESA** (contribution-based)

- **Income-related ESA** (legacy benefit, being replaced by Universal Credit)

Eligibility (New Style ESA):
- You've paid enough National Insurance contributions in the last 2–3 years

- You're too sick to work

- You have a Fit Note

What do you get?
- Around £84.80/week for 13 weeks (the assessment phase)
- After 13 weeks, if you're placed in the Support Group, it increases

How to apply:
- Online or by phone
- You'll need your National Insurance number, GP details, and recent employment history

Necessary: Keep a record of dates, forms, and phone calls. Assume at least one thing will go missing.

Universal Credit (UC): The Necessary Evil

Universal Credit is meant to simplify everything. In practice, it replaces six old benefits and requires you to juggle a clunky website, baffling terminology, and at least one identity verification meltdown.

Who can apply?
- Employed, self-employed, unemployed or too sick to work
- Must have a low income or savings under £16,000

What you might get:
- Standard allowance (depending on age and circumstances)
- Housing support (rent)
- Extra for children or if you're a carer

- **Limited Capability for Work (LCW/LCWRA)** add-on if you're too sick to work

Medical assessment required
- You'll be sent a UC50 form—fill it in like your life depends on it (because it does)
- Include symptom diaries, Fit Notes, GP letters, and real-life examples

Tips for the UC50 form:
- Be brutally honest. Not your best day—your worst.
- Use phrases like: "On most days, I cannot…"
- Explain consequences: "If I do X, I experience severe fatigue and can't function for 2 days."

Sanity-saving advice:
- Take photos of everything you post.
- Expect delays. Be persistent.
- Get help from Citizens Advice or local support groups.

Personal Independence Payment (PIP)
PIP is designed for people who struggle with daily living or mobility. It's not means-tested and can be claimed whether you're working or not.

It's made up of two parts:
1. Daily Living (help with washing, dressing, cooking, etc.)

2. Mobility (difficulty walking or navigating journeys)

You can get one or both parts at standard or enhanced rates.

The Dreaded PIP Form (PIP2)
- 30+ pages of confusing, repetitive questions
- Focus on what you can't do reliably, repeatedly, or safely
- Back up every answer with examples and evidence

Assessment:
- May be face-to-face, phone or video
- Don't "power through" to be polite—describe your real, daily reality

Common question traps:
- "Can you walk 20 metres?" means 20 metres *reliably, safely, in under 2 minutes,* and *without pain or exhaustion.*

If you're refused:
- Ask for a "Mandatory Reconsideration" (MR) within 1 month
- If that fails, appeal to a tribunal—it's often worth it

General Survival Tips for the Bureaucratic Maze

Keep a Symptoms Diary
- Track fatigue, crashes, brain fog, mobility, and pain
- Useful for benefit forms and GP appointments

Photocopy Everything
- Print, scan, save to cloud—don't trust a single envelope

Use Advocates Where Possible
- Citizens Advice, Welfare Rights, disability charities
- They know the tricks of the system

Don't Understate Your Struggle
- This is not the time to be brave or stoic
- Be factual, specific, and real

Brace for Reassessments
- PIP can be awarded for 1, 3 or 10 years
- Keep records even when awarded—future-you will thank you

The Emotional Cost

The benefit system is not kind. It's not built for fluctuating conditions. It rewards clarity and consistency, things Long Covid laughs in the face of.

Expect to feel angry, humiliated, and exhausted. That doesn't mean you're doing it wrong; it means the system needs fixing.

Take breaks. Celebrate small wins—rant to safe people.

You are not a fraud. You are not asking for too much. You are surviving the hardest thing and trying to stay afloat.

And that's worth more than any form will ever reflect.

The Emotional Toll of Financial Strain

Money stress is real. It impacts your mental health, your sleep, and your relationships. It chips away at your sense of autonomy and dignity.

One day, you're managing your mortgage. Next, you're debating whether to spend your last ten quid on paracetamol or dinner.

That emotional whiplash? It's real. And it's allowed to piss you off.

But you are not a failure. You are doing your best in a system that often demands more than it gives. And that deserves recognition, not shame.

> **Your Friend on the Sofa**
>
> You didn't choose to be sick. You didn't choose to have your financial security yanked out from under you. And you shouldn't have to prove your worth to get basic support.
>
> But in this often brutal system, your survival is an act of quiet rebellion.
>
> So track your wins, no matter how small. Claim what you're entitled to. Ask for what you need. And remember: your bank balance does not reflect your value.
>
> You are more than what you earn. You are more than what you owe.
>
> You are worthy – always.

Part Eight - Summary for the Foggy

- Chronic illness drains your **energy *and* your money**.

- Illness brings **unexpected costs**: meds, utilities, food, transport, equipment.

- Work becomes harder—or impossible—leading to **income loss** and career hits.

- **Benefits systems** are complex, slow, and not made for fluctuating conditions.

- Surviving financially means tracking spending, knowing your rights, and asking for help.

- The **emotional toll** is huge—but **you're not weak, you're surviving**.

"This virus left my energy levels lower than my standards during lockdown."

A Last Word From Your Friend On The Sofa

Hope isn't pretending everything's fine. It's not slapping on a smile while your body feels like a phone stuck at 3% battery, even after charging all night. It's not chirpy slogans or being told to "just manifest better vibes."

Real hope is quieter. More grounded. And much, much braver.

It's knowing that things *might* get better—not instantly, not magically, but eventually. Researchers are still in the lab, not giving up. That patient voices are getting louder, and some people- the ones who matter—are finally listening. It's the possibility that your fog might lift. Or thin. Or at least settle into something you can learn to steer through with snacks and noise-cancelling headphones.

Hope doesn't ignore reality. It pulls a chair beside it and says, "Okay, this is where we're at. Let's breathe here a minute."

Some days, hope might look like getting out of bed. Other days, it's choosing to stay in it with a good podcast and clean sheets. Hope is making a tiny plan. Then, rewrite it when your body disagrees and do not beat yourself up for that. Hope is remembering that progress isn't linear. Sometimes it loops. Sometimes it naps.

And if you're surrounded by voices insisting you need to "be positive" or "try harder" or "think yourself better," please know: **that's not hope.** That's marketing. Hope doesn't demand that you smile through the pain.

Hope just quietly says, *You're doing your best. And that's enough.*

You are not broken. You are adapting. You are navigating one of the most complex and misunderstood experiences a human can face—and you're still here.

I'm still trying, loving, and noticing small things, like the weird little bird strutting outside your window with absolute confidence.

You are still very much worth rooting for.

So go forth (or stay put—either is valid).

Rest well.

Laugh loudly, even if it makes you cough a bit.

Pace wisely.

Say no without guilt.

Say yes without pressure.

And maybe, just maybe, enjoy the pigeon show outside your window. They've got the vibe right: a little scruffy, weirdly proud, totally unbothered.

And if you can't hope today, that's okay, I'll hold it for you until you can again.

ABOUT THE AUTHOR

A**lexia Daniels** is a nurse and writer based on the picturesque south coast of England. Her debut novel, *The House of Light & Air*, is the first in a captivating series of historical novels set in the theatres of England, where drama on stage is often rivaled by secrets behind the curtain. Alexia's love for storytelling and history intertwines with her sharp sense of observation—skills honed through her work in healthcare.

Her latest release, *La Vida Loco*, is a deeply personal book born from her experience of Long Covid. Irreverent, honest, and unexpectedly funny, it's the book she never thought she'd write—a no-holds-barred look at chronic illness through the eyes of someone utterly fed up with it.

Her next book, *Sweet Murder*, a witty and twist-filled comedy mystery, is set for release in 2026. Alexia is a proud member of the Portsmouth Author's Collective, where she enjoys connecting with fellow writers and sharing the journey of bringing stories to life.

Thank You

First of all, to **my mum**, who has always been there—through the tears, the multitudinous clerical cock-ups, the copious amounts of coffee, and the many, many rants. You never once told me to "just think positive," and for that alone, you are a hero.

To my friends, who somehow made chronic illness *almost* bearable (a miracle in itself). Whether it was memes, messages, or showing up with snacks and no expectation of conversation—thank you. You laughed with me when I couldn't stand up, and that's real friendship.

My work colleagues—you beautiful humans. Thank you for your kindness, your support, and for not blinking when I showed up looking like a ghost who'd lost a fight with a laundry basket. You kept me going.

Lynn From Devine Designs who created this wonderful cover. It made and continues to make me smile.

A massive thank you to **Dr H in Cardiology**, who casually dropped, "Maybe you should write a book," into conversation and then made me cry (in a good way!) by saying, *"It will get* better. "That moment stuck with me. You gave me hope and on that day I went home and started writing this book.

To the **NHS Long Covid Team**, your work is tireless and your care unshakeable. You are the unsung heroes in a stormy sea of symptoms, acronyms, and baffling fatigue.

Special thanks to **Leah from the NHS Long Covid Vocational Team**—my personal cheerleader, motivator, and the reason the chapter *"Making a Noise"* exists. You reminded me that advocacy is power, and you gave me a voice when I wasn't sure I had one left. Told you I'd write a book.

And finally, to the **Long Covid warriors** out there, especially those putting content out on social media: your honesty, humour, and solidarity are lifelines. When you're stuck on the couch wondering where your life went, finding someone else saying *"same"* can be enough to keep going.

This book is for you.

Even if I never intended to write it.

Even if it's slightly unhinged.

Especially because of that.

Glossary

Mitochondria
The Powerhouse of the Cell™, as every biology teacher has screamed into the void since time began. These microscopic beans turn your food into usable energy (ATP), but in Long Covid? They might be running on dial-up, leaving you feeling like a phone with 3% battery and no charger in sight.

Brain Fog
A charmingly vague term for memory glitches, cognitive slowness, and general mental fuzziness. Like your brain took a personal day but forgot to notify you.

CBT (Cognitive Behavioural Therapy)
A structured, goal-oriented therapy that helps untangle your inner monologue. Great for mental health, anxiety, and processing trauma. Just don't let anyone sell it as a "cure" for your multisystem biomedical condition.

Dysautonomia

When your autonomic nervous system (the one in charge of "auto-pilot" functions like heart rate, digestion, and temperature control) says, "Nope," and starts running on chaos. Common symptoms: dizziness, racing heart, stomach drama, and new respect for standing up.

Energy Envelope

Your personal activity budget. Go over it—say, by walking, thinking too hard, or daring to shower—and you'll trigger PEM. Think of it as an invisible dog fence for your stamina.

ME/CFS (Myalgic Encephalomyelitis/ Chronic Fatigue Syndrome)

A complex, chronic illness that's like Long Covid's older, exhausted cousin. Features include soul-sucking fatigue, PEM, brain fog, and the uncanny ability to confuse doctors since the '80s.

PEM (Post-Exertional Malaise)

A tragic sequel to doing too much. You do a Thing. Hours (or a day) later, your body launches a full-system protest complete with fatigue, pain, and fog. Unlike regular tiredness, PEM feels like you've been hit by a small existential crisis.

POTS (Postural Orthostatic Tachycardia Syndrome)

A form of dysautonomia where standing up sends your heart rate into a panic spiral. Bonus features: nausea, dizziness, and the feeling you've just run a marathon because you reached for the remote.

Pacing

The noble art of doing less—even less than that. It's the opposite of hustle culture. The goal is to avoid triggering symptoms, but the reality feels like negotiating with a grumpy, invisible boss who hates ambition.

Spoon Theory

A metaphor chronic illness warriors swear by. You only get a limited number of spoons (units of energy) each day. Want to shower? That's a spoon. Make lunch? Another one gone. Socialise? Hope you budgeted. Use too many and tomorrow's toast.

Microclots

Tiny, sneaky blood clots that may block capillaries and mess with oxygen delivery. Found in some Long Covid patients. Not big enough to cause classic clots—but just annoying enough to ruin everything quietly.

Inflammatory Soup

Not a menu item, sadly. Refers to the simmering stew of immune system chaos, cytokines, and inflammation sloshing around in some Long Covid bodies. May contribute to brain fog, fatigue, and general "why do I feel like roadkill?" syndrome.

Neuroinflammation

When your brain's immune cells get overexcited and cause swelling or dysfunction. Think of it as brain static. Linked to brain fog, headaches, and why the word you need is *always* on the tip of your tongue.

Relapsing-Remitting

The rollercoaster lifestyle. You feel better for awhile (yay!) and think maybe you're healing... then crash back down (boo). The body's way of keeping your hopes in check.

Orthostatic Intolerance

A fancy way of saying "I can't stand up without turning into a sweaty, dizzy, slightly panicked jellyfish." Seen in POTS, dysautonomia, and that moment in line at the grocery store when you suddenly need to sit *now*.

Useful Stuff - Resources

NHS Long Covid Support
https://www.nhs.uk/conditions/coronavirus-Covid-19/long-term-effects-of-coronavirus-long-Covid/

Your Covid Recovery
https://www.yourCovidrecovery.nhs.uk

Long Covid Support Charity
https://www.longCovid.org

ME Association (for overlapping symptoms with ME/CFS)
https://www.meassociation.org.uk

Action for ME
https://www.actionforme.org.uk

Disability Rights UK
https://www.disabilityrightsuk.org

Equality Advisory and Support Service (EASS)
https://www.equalityadvisoryservice.com

This is just a starter. Have a look and see what works for you.

Useful Stuff - Fit Note Letter

Dear [GP Name],

I am writing to request a fit note in support of ongoing symptoms related to Long Covid, including fatigue, cognitive issues, and Post-Exertional Malaise. These symptoms have impacted my ability to [work/perform daily activities], and I am seeking continued medical documentation for my employer.

Thank you for your time and understanding.

Sincerely,

[Your Name]

Useful Stuff - Workplace Adjustment Request Template

Subject: Request for Workplace Adjustments due to Long Covid

Dear [Manager],

I have been managing symptoms of Long Covid, including fatigue and [insert the symptoms which bother you most at work].

I want to discuss possible reasonable adjustments, such as [flexible hours / remote work / longer breaks].

I'm happy to provide documentation or speak with Occupational Health.

I appreciate your support.

Best regards,
[Your Name]

Useful Stuff - Tracker for GP

Medical History Summary – Long COVID
Name:
Date of Birth:
Phone/Email:
Date Updated:

Main Condition

- **Primary diagnosis:** Long COVID / Post-COVID Syndrome

- **Date of COVID-19 infection:**

- **Date of Diagnosis of Long Covid:**

- **Hospitalisation?** ☐ Yes ☐ No

- If yes, duration and level of care:

Current Symptoms
(Check or briefly describe current symptoms)
- ☐ Fatigue(chronic/severe)
- ☐ Brain fog /cognitive issues
- ☐ Shortness of breath
- ☐ Chest pain or palpitations
- ☐ POTS/dizziness
- ☐ Headaches
- ☐ Muscle/joint pain
- ☐ Sleep disturbances
- ☐ GI symptoms
- ☐ Anxiety / low mood
- ☐ Other:_____

Medications& Supplements
Name   Dose   Reason

Key Tests & Results
Test   Date   Result/Notes

Specialists Seen
Specialty   Name / Clinic   Key Notes / Plan

Other Diagnoses or Health Conditions

-
-
-
-

Other Notes or Questions for GP

-
-
-
-

www.ingramcontent.com/pod-product-compliance
Lightning Source LLC
Chambersburg PA
CBHW051529020426
42333CB00016B/1838